D0613766

I DO NOT CONSENT

My Fight Against Medical Cancel Culture

Simone Gold, M.D., J.D.

BOMBARDIER BOOKS
An Imprint of Post Hill Press
ISBN: 978-1-63758-085-1
ISBN (eBook): 978-1-64293-891-3

I Do Not Consent:
My Fight Against Medical Cancel Culture
© 2021 by Simone Gold, M.D., J.D.
All Rights Reserved
Cover art by Tiffani Shea
Cover photo by Breitbart News

This book contains advice and information relating to health care. It should be used to supplement rather than replace the advice of your doctor or another trained health professional. You are advised to consult your health professional with regard to matters related to your health, and in particular regarding matters that may require diagnosis or medical attention. All efforts have been made to assure the accuracy of the information in this book as of the date of publication. The publisher and the author disclaim liability for any medical outcomes that may occur as a result of applying the methods suggested in this book.

No part of this book may be reproduced, stored in a retrieval system, or transmitted by any means without the written permission of the author and publisher.

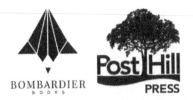

Post Hill Press
New York • Nashville
posthillpress.com

Published in the United States of America

This book is dedicated to my parents and my children. May the chain remain unbroken.

TABLE OF CONTENTS

I.

PATIENT ONE: ON THE FRONTLINES OF THE COVID PANDEMIC

The virus arrived largely without warning, particularly for the general public. As events unfolded, media coverage portrayed a world at war with an invisible combatant. Glowing red blobs superimposed on the map showed the blast radius of infections rippling out from its epicenter in Wuhan—a city in eastern China's Hubei Province and home to China's only level four biosafety lab—then to the industrial north of Italy, on to the rest of Europe, and eventually to population centers on the coasts of the continental United States. We were watching unfold a situation that no one alive had seen or managed. Sure, we read about global viral pandemics in history books and medical journals. But being on the frontlines and dealing with it in real time was a new experience.

COVID-19 is the respiratory disease caused by the new or "novel" human coronavirus. We knew at the time that the pathogen spread through droplets in coughs and sneezes, and that it was highly contagious. Precautions were taken. These included hand-washing, disinfection, and social distancing. Handshakes were out; people avoided large group gatherings when possible. Most important of all, Americans from the boardroom to the corner bodega were told to stay home from work if they felt sick.

My state of California recorded its first case of the virus on January 26, 2020. By February the international body responsible for naming viruses had settled on SARS-SoV-2 owing to its genetic similarities with the class of virus responsible for the Chinese SARS outbreak of 2002. President Trump declared a public health emergency on February 3. Complex geopolitics combined with a naive trust in Chinese health officials led the World Health Organization (WHO) to delay its labeling COVID-19 a global pandemic until almost the middle of March.

In the United States, the disease began as a cluster of infections in a suburban nursing home east of Seattle and resulted in the first U.S. death associated with COVID-19 on February 29. The same day, the U.S. surgeon general admonished Americans for buying face masks, tweeting "Seriously people—stop buying masks! They are not effective in preventing general public [sic] from catching #Coronavirus ...." As new cases and deaths climbed in March, fears of overwhelmed, under-equipped hospitals grew as well.

By mid-March President Trump's administration had issued new guidelines to slow the virus's spread, including avoiding discretionary travel and groups of ten or more people when possible. The media's coverage of the lack of testing supplies intensified. According to a poll released by the American Psychiatric Association, 48 percent of Americans reported that they felt anxious about the possibility of contracting coronavirus. Meanwhile, healthcare workers on the frontlines bore the brunt of the emergency—and the risk.

Then on March 13, President Trump declared a national emergency, directing billions of dollars and a massive intergovernmental effort to contain the spread. Like a majority of Americans in those days, doctors were still unclear what was happening. To the extent the US media commented on COVID-19, its coverage had been uneven and slow to catch up with partisan domestic priorities such as the impeachment and the Mueller report. Elected officials in both parties sent mixed signals based on bad information from the WHO, China, and other sources.

Not long afterwards I started seeing my first COVID patients. The question in my mind was how to provide the most effective care given the uncertainty of the moment.

My colleagues were placing virtually every symptomatic person they saw on oxygen and treating most with antibiotics. These patients had their heartbeats monitored as well.

The common antimalarial drug called hydroxychloroquine (HCQ) had been shown to be effective against the first SARS outbreak close to two decades ago. Could it work now, I wondered? I knew about HCQ because many years ago when I was planning a trip to Africa, the travel physician just handed me the prescription—no conversation—just, "Here, take this, start now." It was a simple, white tablet, taken weekly. The drug can be safely taken by pregnant women and nursing mothers, the young and the old.

My personal experience with the drug coupled with my physician's knowledge that it's extremely safe meant I was excited about its treatment possibilities for COVID-19. The U.K.'s Imperial College COVID Response Team had recently predicted more than two million Americans could die if no actions were taken. HCQ was something I could use to treat patients right away in an emerging situation.

My first confirmed positive patient was a woman in her fifties in the mid-stages of COVID-19. When I saw her in the emergency department of the hospital where I worked, her symptoms included a low fever and some shortness of breath with chest pain, but otherwise she was stable. The woman was somewhat sick and faced a significant chance of becoming critically ill, but at the moment she was in pretty good shape. She could take medications on her own, had a family prepared to monitor her progress, and could return if her condition worsened. She was the perfect outpatient candidate for hydroxychloroquine. Let's call her Patient One.

In the early days of the pandemic, people were innovating and trying new things. For example, by late March the FDA was letting doctors apply to administer convalescent plasma—the antibody-rich blood drawn from COVID-recovered individuals—to their patients on a case-by-case basis. They pointed out that plasma had been an effective treatment for other coronaviruses. I saw HCQ in much the same way. Early-adopter physicians like me were intrigued by the potential of HCQ. The opposing opinion was simply "do what you think is best." At this point there was no controversy.

I saw both in- and outpatients at the time. Inpatients are those requiring hospitalization while outpatients can be discharged from the emergency department. Unlike the experience at some hospitals, equipment shortages fortunately never became an issue in ours. We had enough personal protective equipment (PPE) for the nurses and doctors.

I had done my residency training in New York and I quizzed my former colleagues during the early days of COVID-19. I read all the available clinical studies and followed the administration's daily Coronavirus Task Force briefings when I wasn't working clinically. As physicians, we were extremely conscientious about personal protective equipment. We were very careful about going home and possibly bringing the virus with us. We talked among ourselves almost compulsively about the availability of masks because we were the doctors doing the highest-risk procedures—intubations—inserting a tube into a patient's trachea in order to open an airway for oxygen or medication.

In preparing to treat Patient One I had followed Dr. Didier Raoult's studies from Marseilles, France, the early studies from China, and those of a clinician named Dr. Zev Zelenko from New York, who had himself treated many hundreds of patients. Dr. Raoult had documented his success in treating COVID patients with HCQ at his clinic in southern France. Dr. Zelenko tested the drug regimen thousands of us would go on to prescribe.

Dr. Harvey Risch, M.D., Ph.D., professor of epidemiology at the Yale School of Public Health, authored the most comprehensive study published on HCQ to date. It reviewed five outpatient studies, including Raoult's, dealing with hydroxychloroquine and demonstrated how they had been either misinterpreted or willfully misreported in the media. I had also been tracking the worldwide scientific literature on HCQ. The most common side effect is mild nausea. According to US Centers for Disease Control and Prevention (CDC) research, "chloroquine [an earlier analog of HCQ] has been widely used to treat human diseases, such as malaria, amoebiasis, HIV, and autoimmune diseases, without significant detrimental side effects."

HCQ was a drug which I knew had had billions of dosages (just in America) since the FDA approved it in April 1955. Decades of medical studies had proved its safety over and over again, and the vast majority of recent studies favored its effectiveness against COVID. Clinical guidance suggested by studies of HCQ indicate that as a treatment it's more effective to use at the onset of illness rather than after hospitalization for COVID. This made it all the more likely to be useful to someone like me, who would typically see patients presenting with medium- and early-onset symptoms.

Some of my colleagues were skeptical; most were indifferent. I didn't share their premises. I had done my homework. As far as I was concerned, hydroxychloroquine worked, and at worst would do no harm.

I recommended this "off-label" treatment to Patient One as an antiviral therapy. Drug "repositioning" or "off-label use" is a common practice in which medications used for certain existing diseases are repurposed as treatments for others. I prescribed a combination of HCQ, an antibiotic called azithromycin, and zinc. Zinc deficiency frequently occurs in elderly patients and in those with cardiovascular disease. The lower the zinc levels, the easier it is for COVID-19 to reproduce itself inside a host.

I discharged Patient One the same day with instructions to follow up. Within twenty-four hours her condition dramatically improved. HCQ and zinc suppressed the viral replication in her body and the patient rapidly got better. The literature and the doctors I followed had been right! Innovation backed by scientific evidence had helped her. I was thrilled.

The day after I got the good news about Patient One, the hospital's medical director called.

He told me he learned that I had prescribed hydroxychloroquine to an outpatient. That statement in and of itself was highly unusual. He was the administrative director, but doctors practice independently and no one checks the prescribing practice of one's peers.

I couldn't believe my ears. This felt like an interrogation.

I had successfully treated a sick patient in the midst of a national emergency with a reliable drug. He began by insisting the drug "wasn't indicated," and that in his opinion he didn't think its use was justified.

I had been challenged by people before. My mind returned to medical school in Chicago. I had graduated college at nineteen and was the youngest in my medical school class—just a "kid." My age and gender influenced how people reacted to my medical analysis. Just like those school days, though, I was determined to succeed by believing in myself and working hard. But this wasn't about sexism or ageism. It was different. For one thing, the director's criticism lacked basic logic and ignored science.

So I did what any doctor should do: I countered with facts. "Well, it's not indicated for inpatients either," I said, referencing those too sick to discharge. Three weeks earlier the hospital had begun administering HCQ to those already hospitalized. It was safe and effective for inpatients but forbidden for outpatients, according to his line of argument. One day it was not indicated, the next it was. "In two weeks you'll say to me it is indicated," I added. This was the first interaction of its kind I had had with this medical director. It made no sense.

A potentially lethal virus was spreading in California. The hospital had treated an infected patient with a common, safe, effective drug and she recovered. I had expected to get kudos. Instead I was met with hostility. The severity of the response was bizarre. And the sudden interest in my prescribing practice was unprecedented.

He flat-out told me I was irritating the powerful consortium affiliated with our hospital, the largest of its kind in the United States encompassing hospitals, medical clinics, and administrative offices in this part of California for three-quarters of a century. Why would this be the case? Regardless, it seemed that the business of medicine was taking priority over the practice of patient care. The conversation ended when the medical director basically said he would fire me if I ever gave HCQ to an outpatient again.

It was the strangest encounter I had ever had with a medical colleague. It came seemingly out of nowhere, almost as though an alien force had taken control of him—like something out of the 1950s film *Invasion of the Body Snatchers*. Unfortunately, it wouldn't be the last.

It's one thing for the public at large to blindly follow someone on television who seems to know something. But to see physicians voluntarily surrender their medical judgment was positively surreal.

I've been a part of the medical profession since before ~~I was born. My father was a doctor and my mother and~~ grandmother handled the billing and managed the practice. My father saw his patients in hospitals and nursing homes all day and held office hours every evening at our home. He never took a vacation, almost never took a day off, and told me every day that I would be a doctor. Medicine is an inseparable part of my identity. It's who I am.

For most of my career I have chosen to serve residents of the inner city. I have always worked with the poor and underserved. It is a very difficult job. Anyone who wants to know what socialized medicine would look like in this country need look no further than their local emergency room. I tell my friends and family to avoid the emergency department (ED) at almost any cost. While the doctors, nurses, tech and administrative staff at EDs tend to be outstanding individuals, the healthcare system as a whole is so broken that it's harmful. More often than not, due to government interference at every level of the process, it takes a herculean effort to do the right thing. I have to over-test, over-treat, over-order, overcompensate, under-think, under-feel, and under-serve just to get past the rules that well-intentioned but inflexible bureaucrats have put in place to "protect" the patient.

These dynamics went into high gear when, on March 19, President Trump, standing alongside his Coronavirus Task Force, called HCQ a "game changer." On March 21, President Trump tweeted a message about HCQ paired with azithromycin. The FDA issued an emergency-use authorization for chloroquine phosphate and hydroxychloroquine sulfate for tens of millions of doses from the Strategic National Stockpile on March 28.

That's when the elite media, the medical establishment, their allies in the political world, and the social media mob launched their war against a humble malaria drug. Headline after headline falsely called the treatment untested, unproven, and worse. On March 21 Bloomberg News told readers that "evidence is lacking" for HCQ's effectiveness. The Financial Times in an April 13 headline speculated that HCQ might be a "dangerous gamble." Also, in the UK, the Guardian newspaper warned its audience, "don't believe the hype."

On March 20, a day after Trump mentioned the drug, Dr. Anthony Fauci, the powerful and media-savvy director of the National Institute of Allergy and Infectious Diseases (NIAID), answered "no" when asked if he thought HCQ had promise. "[T]he evidence you're talking about … is anecdotal evidence," he said.

Never mind that the treatment's safe and effective use has been voluminously documented in leading medical journals over sixty-five years. HCQ was only subject to a shifting consensus in the days and weeks after Donald Trump publicly acknowledged its use as an effective treatment. All of a sudden, HCQ was regarded as dangerous snake oil hawked by quacks and charlatans instead of a proven and efficacious treatment routinely prescribed by doctors and available over the counter in many parts of the world for decades.

Our department's team consisted of thirty or so physicians and advanced practice providers (APP)—a group of nurse practitioners and physician assistants. Soon we got the new molecular diagnostic coronavirus testing kits that provided results in under an hour. This made testing and treating people easier.

I kept on prescribing hydroxychloroquine and zinc as a COVID-19 treatment to the confirmed-positive cases I saw. Over the next six weeks I treated around ten patients with HCQ. Just like my first case, their conditions improved. The "anecdotal evidence" that some people mocked wasn't anecdotal to me. It was someone's wife, someone's brother, someone's uncle, someone's father.

Although I didn't push or proselytize the treatment to other doctors, I knew of two in my own group who agreed with me. I also knew many others who stockpiled the drug. On the flip side, one physician in my group managed to never have an independent thought—he literally changed his opinion whenever Dr. Fauci changed his. To me, this was another *Body Snatchers* moment.

Then came a sudden and nonsensical reversal. The CDC announced on April 7 that there were no approved drugs to treat COVID-19. "Hydroxychloroquine and chloroquine are under investigation in clinical trials" for use on coronavirus patients and "there are no drugs or other therapeutics approved by the US Food and Drug Administration to prevent or treat COVID-19," the agency's updated guidelines stated. It was downright bizarre to single out HCQ like this, I thought. I began to suspect some kind of behind-the-scenes decision had been made to sideline the drug.

In May, the other shoe dropped. Very suddenly, "respectable" research papers were rapidly published claiming HCQ was ineffective at treating COVID-19 and dangerous. *The Lancet*, a British medical journal, linked HCQ with heartbeat irregularities as part of a dubious study that was later discredited. Nevertheless, changes at my hospital followed.

The Lancet's study tracked over ninety thousand patients, concluding that HCQ decreased hospital survival rates and increased heartbeat irregularity that could be dangerous in certain people. HCQ was being blamed for patient deaths.

Immediately, the World Health Organization announced that it would be suspending clinical trials being held in hundreds of hospitals across the world, the European health ministers of France, Italy, Belgium, and other EU members banned HCQ for COVID-19 trials, and it ordered nations to stop using HCQ. The American press had a field day mocking the president and others who had backed HCQ as a treatment: "Study of Trump-touted chloroquine for coronavirus stopped due to heart problems, deaths," blared the April 15 headline of USA Today. "Trump Says He's Taking Hydroxychloroquine, Prompting Warning From Health Experts," the New York Times informed its readership on May 18. "His announcement drew immediate criticism from a range of medical experts, who warned not just of the dangers it posed for the president's health but also of the example it set," the paper wrote.

I smelled something fishy. How did *The Lancet* study researchers get more than ninety thousand patients' data from hundreds of hospitals analyzed and published so quickly? And why was the lead researcher the only author to have seen the raw numbers?

My hunch was right: as it turned out, *The Lancet* study was a fake. The fraudulent research, highlighted by my future colleague in America's Frontline Doctors, Dr. James Todaro, was carried out by a tiny company called Surgisphere based in Chicago. At the time of the research in question, Surgisphere had only six employees, including a science fiction writer and another billing herself as an adult model and events hostess, according to their website, which has since been scrubbed from the internet.

Independent physicians demanded that the authors independently verify the patient data—a requirement of being published in *The Lancet*. The authors refused, likely because no such data even existed. Less than two weeks after its findings went public, *The Lancet* retracted its HCQ study. A retraction of such significance is nearly unheard of in this field, occurring perhaps once in a generation. The retraction and corruption of the research was never given the same attention in the press or online as the original study blasting HCQ. The public therefore was at best confused, or at worst relying on junk science.

Around the same time as the disgraced *Lancet* report, a study in *The New England Journal of Medicine* was published also using Surgisphere patient data to observe the treatment effects of HCQ. This too was retracted after NEJM admitted it could not account for the underlying research. But the retractions hardly mattered as they were again poorly publicized and the damage to the public's perception of HCQ had already been done.

After *The Lancet* and *The New England Journal of Medicine* studies appeared, I noticed two categories of physicians: those who said HCQ wasn't safe, and those who said it wasn't effective. It seemed that my colleagues were suddenly no longer interested in either thinking for themselves or using their critical judgment to get the best possible outcome for patients.

This was not a dispute over the merits of the academic literature. Those disagreements happen frequently. Only a couple of weeks earlier my medical group had had a conversation (some might call it a spirited debate) about the relative merits of using epinephrine—also known as adrenaline—for advanced cardiopulmonary resuscitation patients on life support. Getting into the nitty gritty was a normal and natural part of working in the emergency department. Not anymore. Independent thinkers had been replaced by risk-averse technocrats taking orders from the government, the consortium, even the media.

Washington figures like Nancy Pelosi lined up against HCQ on the incredible grounds that it was "something that has not been approved by scientists," and added that the drug wasn't intended for the likes of the "morbidly obese" President Trump. The issue was being completely politicized and average Americans were being forced to pick a side. An April survey of registered voters showed 65 percent of Democrats would not use the drug; meanwhile, 71 percent of Republicans supported the treatment.

As the reputation of HCQ declined, the emergency powers granted to governors by their state legislatures were increasingly being abused. In Michigan, when Republicans refused to go along with extending Democratic Governor Gretchen Whitmer's stay-at-home order closing businesses and restricting her citizen's movements, the governor simply enacted a new order unilaterally. Similarly in my state of California, Governor Gavin Newsom used a March 19 mandatory quarantine order to keep beaches and outdoor events shut down despite a flurry of lawsuits.

From the federal government down to the local level, it was worrisome to me to watch the lockstep conformity of those listening to the CDC's public pronouncements and the media's spin. This just wasn't the way doctors practiced medicine, I thought. In my decades-long experience treating patients in hospital settings, I couldn't recall a single conversation with colleagues which began, "Let's see what the CDC says to do and then do that." Our decisions were influenced by our education and formal training, experience, articles in scientific journals, and discussions with colleagues. To us, the CDC was less than irrelevant: it was nonexistent. I was witnessing a sea change, and I didn't like what I saw.

There was a total absence of debate grounded in science and evidence. It was like watching prime-time cable news: all opinion and no facts. Doctors I worked alongside claimed to be "following the science" in their aversion to prescribing hydroxychloroquine. The reality was different. I had been tracking the worldwide scientific literature on HCQ. The medical studies proved its safety over and over again, and the vast majority favored its effectiveness as well. I was actually working in an area that was more red than blue politically and it did not feel as though partisan politics was relevant. We doctors certainly never talked politics or discussed what a politician thought. It was simply that *The Lancet* or the CDC was right and that was that.

Suddenly a collective hysteria seemed to grip the scientific-medical establishment. The prohibition against HCQ contradicted everything I had learned about medicine since I worked as a young intern. Prior to March 2020, every doctor all over the world knew HCQ was safe. It is the most commonly prescribed drug in India, the second-most populous nation in the world. In much of the world it is sold next to vitamin C or D in the vitamin section of any ordinary shop. Thousands of doctors across the globe attested to its effectiveness in treating COVID-19. I personally experienced its effectiveness, and most of my peers also knew at least one physician who knew it worked.

I concluded that the majority of doctors simply felt they needed to keep their heads down, and that's much easier to do if you don't think too hard about what you are doing.

I could see that our politicized and biased media coverage, as well as the corruption of key scientific studies, meant most patients in America would not get properly treated if hydroxychloroquine were prescription-only. I knew that we needed to make this drug widely available—bypassing doctors, pharmacists, and tyrannical governors—by making it available over the counter like it is in most of the world.

Sadly, our inaction has had dire consequences. Many in the media and politics blame the Trump administration for letting (as of this writing) some two hundred thousand Americans die of COVID-19. Few of them seem willing to consider the more immediate and certain truth: if HCQ had not been blocked from distribution by shadowy forces, both private and political, whose role and motivations are still not known or clearly understood, far fewer people would have died. Countries where HCQ is widely available have orders of magnitude fewer deaths than Western nations—and the American anti-HCQ media still denies that HCQ is the reason. "Coincidence" they call it. "Anecdotal" they say. Eighty positive studies later and their minds still haven't changed.

But I was never one to go along. Not in college, not in med school; not in my days as a law student at Stanford. I wasn't about to start now.

Little did I know that, as a frontline emergency physician speaking about what I had personally observed, Big Tech would work overtime to censor me and Big Media would go into hyper-overdrive to defame me.

II.

WHY I SPOKE OUT ABOUT HCQ—AND WHAT HAPPENED NEXT

One afternoon in July, in the midst of the pandemic, I stood in the thick heat of a Washington, D.C., summer, with concerned physicians from around the country in front of the US Supreme Court and proclaimed my independence from the medical cancel culture. "We're America's Frontline Doctors," I began. Camera shutters clicked energetically around the eighteen or so experienced physicians gathered at the high court's majestic west front facade. "We're here only to help American patients and the American nation heal," I continued. Then I laid out the facts as I had come to know them firsthand through my E.R. work: that before you get the virus or in the early stages of infection, there is treatment.

The event was digitally livestreamed as part of my daylong "White Coat Summit" organized by our relatively unknown yet growing collective, America's Frontline Doctors. In a year of unprecedented change for virtually all of us who care about this profession, my biggest 2020 transformation would find me three thousand miles from work, family, and home, fighting to speak the unvarnished truth about fighting the pandemic in our nation's capital.

What brought me there? For this story, we have to turn back the clock to four demanding months of disappointment and hope.

In an unusual joint statement on April 17, 2020, the American Medical Association, along with the American Pharmacists Association and American Society of Health-System Pharmacists, issued the following warning to practicing doctors like me:

> [W]e caution hospitals, health systems, other entities, and individual practitioners that no medication has been FDA-approved for use in COVID-19 patients. Definitive evidence for the role of these drugs in treating COVID-19 patients has not been determined through robust clinical trials; decisions to use these medications off-label must be made with extreme caution and careful monitoring. Physicians, pharmacists, patients and policymakers

must understand that these medications have dangerous side effects that may lead to patient harm, including fatal cardiac arrhythmias.

I knew this wasn't so. Since at least 2005 there was also evidence in the medical literature that hydroxychloroquine was effective in treating human coronavirus because of its repositioning as a SARS drug. The best dispassionate explanation correcting the "big lie" that HCQ was not safe before turning to the drug's efficacy was published by Yale's Dr. Harvey Risch.

First, Dr. Risch pointed out that early evidence supporting HCQ's record of safety was ignored: "Lack of any cardiac arrhythmia events in the 405 Zelenko patients or the 1,061 Marseilles patients or the 412 Brazil patients." Next, Risch noticed correctly that safety concerns among the large public health institutions seem to be driven by something other than science: namely, partisan politics. "It is unclear why the FDA, NIH, and cardiology societies made their [negative] recommendations about HCQ+AZM now, when the Oxford study analyzed 323,122 users of HCQ+AZ ... that the combination of HCQ+AZM has been in widespread standard-of-care use in the US and elsewhere for decades ... this use being predominantly in older adults with multiple comorbidities, with no such strident warnings about the use given during that time," he wrote.

In his defense of the drug's effectiveness, Risch noted that Dr. Raoult's pro-HCQ study in France was criticized for its lack of a randomized controlled trial. At the time,

Raoult responded to his critics by invoking what is known as the parachute paradigm. Put simply, parachutes reduce harm. This has come to be accepted despite the fact that no study was ever produced in which an experimental parachute faced off against a control group of jumpers with no parachutes. Likewise, if a treatment for infectious disease "works" as it should, the result ought to be visible to anyone observing it, perhaps immediately. But you've got to jump first in order to find out.

Dr. Risch, with almost forty thousand Google Scholar citations to his credit—as many as the National Institute of Allergy and Infectious Diseases Director, Dr. Anthony Fauci—sided with Raoult.

The AMA had put its considerable thumb on the scale and come out against prescribing hydroxychloroquine—a drug which I knew to be safe and effective in treating COVID-19. The voice of the scientific-medical establishment had spoken, and once again many of my colleagues had simply fallen in line, not wanting to buck the medical establishment or those who have outsized influence over it. Though I was on friendly terms with many of these doctors, I would soon be forced to recalibrate my view of them.

I thought back to the last pandemic threat several years earlier and the yawning gap between the severity of the crisis and the underwhelming response. What played out then was virtually the opposite of today's COVID controversy.

At the time of the 2014 Ebola outbreak threat, the lethal illness had been carried to other countries from West

Africa mostly by medical workers. A patient in Dallas, Texas, had already died from the disease and a medical aid volunteer was hospitalized with symptoms in New York City after returning from Guinea. I was working as an emergency physician in Inglewood, California, the low-income, gang-ridden, majority-minority city that provided the setting for the tough 1991 drama *Boyz N the Hood*. Due to our facility's short distance from LAX, we were designated to be the receiving hospital for any potential Ebola cases in our part of the state. After the CDC confirmed its first case in late 2014, our hospital started Ebola training protocols.

I couldn't believe that this was the plan. "You know what I'm going to do when an Ebola patient comes off the plane to our hospital?" I asked the other doctors and nurses. "I'm leaving and I suggest you do too." They paused and stared, not comprehending.

I continued: "There's something fundamentally wrong with the system when someone with Ebola is allowed to fly seven thousand miles and be transported to our totally ill-equipped E.R. to expose all the doctors and nurses, ancillary staff, and other patients who happened to show up that day to a highly contagious, nearly always rapidly fatal, horrific hemorrhagic disease. That's not our fault—there's something wrong with the CDC deciding we all should possibly die for their failures."

Instead of the agency using its personnel in West Africa to contain Ebola before it was allowed to spread, the CDC's patchwork approach routed at-risk passengers to screening airports like LAX with the intention of sending positive cases to my hospital.

At the end of the day, I did not care what their reasons were. I was not letting my fellow doctors and nurses possibly die because there was a woefully inadequate response by public health experts on a global scale, including my own country. My colleagues were not going to be guinea pigs for failed Washington politicians or policies. Let the cowardly CDC doctors who were passing the buck come take care of such patients, I thought. It was easy for them to order others to take grave risks while they were kept safely out of harm's way. To this day, I will never forget that it was the CDC who so obviously considered frontline doctors, nurses, and supporting staff expendable.

Our government's decision to send an ill-equipped community hospital in a poor black neighborhood a lethal disease from seven thousand miles away was an eye-opening moment for me. It showed me how easily governments and the scientific community could do the wrong thing. Now I saw it happening again. HCQ's promise as an effective treatment was being ignored. Bureaucrats were drawing on bad science in order to tell doctors what to do, and average Americans were put at risk.

On April 24, 2020, the Journal of the American Medical Association, the mouthpiece of the nation's foremost health organization, published a study on chloroquine that turned out to be patently reckless—if not criminal.

Right off the bat, something didn't look right about this supposedly airtight study's methodology.

The study was led by a clinical researcher in Brazil starting in March, when COVID cases were growing steadily in the research team's part of the country. Brazil's government had touted HCQ—widely available there as an antimalarial drug—as a treatment for hospitalized patients and was debating expanding its use to outpatients at the time the experiments were conducted.

A group of older, sicker, hospitalized participants in the clinical trial were given toxic amounts of chloroquine, contradicting basic medical practice with the drug. More than thirty years earlier, the lethal dose of CQ was established as five grams. A four-gram dose on its own was linked to severe neurological and cardiovascular toxicity. JAMA's high-dose group received 4.8 grams in just four days and twelve grams if they survived to the full ten days of the trial. This is 2.5 times the lethal dose. And in fact, so many people did die in the high-dose group that the experiment had to be halted. Peter Kremsner of the University of Tübingen in Germany, conducting HCQ research of his own, called the Brazilian study's doses "dangerous and definitely too high."

An abnormally high dosage had been deliberately administered to an older, sicker set of patients. Investigators are still trying to understand why. Given decades of standard clinical practice with the drug, what did the study's authors expect to happen? But the official journal of the world's most powerful medical association had spoken. JAMA joined *The New England Journal of Medicine* and *The Lancet* in pushing anti-HCQ bias, but unlike the other two, no retraction has ever come from the JAMA editor. There is, however, ongoing civil and criminal investigations into twenty-seven scientists over the deaths of those patients.

The damage had been done. Based primarily on these flawed studies, the FDA revoked its emergency use authorization (EUA) for HCQ on June 15, dealing advocates for the treatment another crushing blow. The Biomedical Advanced Research and Development Authority (BARDA) was the agency inside the Department of Health and Human Services (HHS) responsible for prodding the FDA to revoke hydroxychloroquine's EUA.

This disconnect between the science and reality appeared to drive internal conflict at HHS when BARDA Director Rick Bright was removed from his post and reassigned to the National Institutes of Health allegedly for clashing with senior department officials over HCQ. He said HCQ was "distracting to dozens of government scientists" at his division, the FDA, and the NIH who were trying to develop COVID-19 vaccines and other treatments. At least someone at HHS disagreed.

Nevertheless, the media had another martyr for their cause. Politicians responded by presenting Dr. Bright as a courageous whistleblower. One lamented that he'd been "fired for being right."

Junk science offered a pretense to certain elements within the scientific-medical establishment to call HCQ ineffective and risky and rein in its use. Soon a consensus about the drug had formed among the highest scientific ranks and spread to interested parties in the government and the media. This consensus then hardened into a prejudice. International bodies like the World Health Organization and the Centre for Evidence-Based Medicine in the UK lined up to deliver their negative verdicts, reinforcing the anti-HCQ narrative.

These announcements were followed by weeks of seemingly coordinated media attacks. It became almost impossible to find any positive news about the drug in US news reports. The mainstream press either ignored the evidence of its effectiveness or buried the findings. There are different sorts of biases, and omission bias—simply not reporting certain things—is now the norm in all media. Omission bias is the most dangerous type of bias because the reader thinks he or she is informed. In fact, you are much worse off for having read "news" with **omission bias.**

For example, at approximately the same time the fraudulent *Lancet*, NEJM and JAMA studies were being heavily promoted and published by the American media, one of the oldest and most reputable medical journals in the world reported that hydroxychloroquine was highly effective for high-risk healthcare workers. This study was simply not reported at all in America. Another example of omission bias is the Detroit study, which the mainstream media published on the Friday before July 4 in an obvious attempt to be unseen by as many as possible. These are just two of over eighty positive studies which received almost no media attention.

Newspapers, cable TV, and especially social media platforms began to resemble nothing less than propaganda outlets from the bad old days of 20th-century dictatorships. Their bias signaled a conscious disrespect for scientific evidence and the judgment of both physicians and the general public.

An important rule in medicine is to follow the scientific evidence, not to act out of fear. The basic reproduction number (known as R or R-naught) is a figure epidemiologists use to measure how fast a virus is spreading. By March 1, California's R was 2.48. This meant that a COVID-infected person was expected to spread the virus, on average, to two and a half additional people. As R goes up, contagiousness and infections rise.

By April into May, no other treatment options were as readily available for a highly contagious virus as hydroxychloroquine taken with azithromycin (AZM) and zinc. With lockdowns and state medical decrees aggressively chipping away at the doctor-patient relationship, governments were now fully invested in the politics of fear. Instead of offering effective medication and treatment—and, most importantly, hope—we were peddling fear and justifying lockdowns. I was deeply dispirited. Yet I knew I had to act.

I also knew I couldn't act alone. I needed a group of passionate, like-minded physicians who had also been blocked from participating in the national debate. After two weeks' worth of legwork and hustle in my very limited free time, I had assembled a large group of other silenced doctors: frontline physicians from many specialties: pediatricians, cardiologists, surgeons, psychiatrists, and more. All of them could attest that the lockdown-cure for coronavirus had been worse than the disease.

On May 19 I sent a letter to the Trump administration to this effect, co-signed by seven hundred other doctors. "It is impossible to overstate the short, medium, and long-term harm to people's health with a continued shutdown," I wrote.

The letter warned of a "mass casualty incident" if business and school-lockdown mandates were left in place much longer. The heartbreaking consequences had already been observed up close and documented by me and countless other physicians: deferred medical treatment, substance abuse, growing rates of depression, and other mental illness. One doctor I knew told me about a patient who was prevented from getting the wound care she required due to the quarantine measures, resulting in the amputation of her leg below the knee. Forty to 50 percent of strokes and heart attacks simply went "missing" compared to data from previous years. My hospitals, just like others all across the country, were nearly empty. Nationwide, hospital staff was furloughed and let go. My physician hours were cut 20 to 30 percent and half of the emergency techs were let go.

My letter was intended as a wake-up call to NIAID's Dr. Fauci. The New Yorker had declared him "America's Doctor." Brad Pitt portrayed Fauci on "Saturday Night Live" as the omnicompetent medical expert with a Brooklyn accent. While average Americans were forced to shelter in place and miss birthdays and funerals, he would go on to land cover shoots in glossy fashion magazines and throw out the first pitch for Major League Baseball. I knew his advice to other Coronavirus Task Force members advocating a nationwide shutdown would inflict real pain on a fearful and anxious public. He led the way in calling HCQ's treatment record anecdotal and unproven.

The letter served as a reminder—with some attention-grabbing phrases—that doctors like Fauci had an obligation to be honest with the public. I felt his pessimistic assessments were doing nothing to teach Americans about balancing risk with quality of life.

Meanwhile, I waited to see what (if anything) would happen in response to my letter. Public advocacy was still a new role for me and I didn't yet understand the ins and outs of Washington. Finally, an answer came back from someone I knew close to the administration. Vice President Pence and others had read our letter. Even better, it seemed that our words had had an effect on public policy: the next day Dr. Fauci reversed his rigid stance on lockdowns, predicting "irreparable damage" if they continued.

After weeks of grassroots organizing efforts, I felt vindicated if not completely satisfied by our recent success.

But I knew that I had to continue my fight.

On May 24 I appeared on television, or rather YouTube, for the first time. A "Reopen California" rally was held in Sacramento at the capitol to protest Governor Newsom's expansive lockdown order in place since March 19 that closed everything from small businesses to houses of worship with fines up to $1,000 for violating the law. I didn't think it was right for the state government to deny people their liberty and freedom for an invalid reason, so I attended the rally and shared my thoughts with a lively crowd of hundreds of independent-minded Americans.

"When I read the stories from doctors, it breaks your heart. There's cancer patients that can't get chemotherapy. Forty percent of stroke victims went missing during the lockdowns. These stories are heartbreaking," I said. I spoke at the rally with radio and internet personality Dennis Prager and Dr. Jeff Barke, a board-certified primary care physician in Orange County.

I never mentioned my emerging policy activism at the hospitals where I worked. I was there to deliver care to patients and my worlds remained deliberately separate. But I had begun seeking out doctors who shared my commitment to science and truth. I wanted Americans to have the ability to make up their own minds about HCQ, the lockdowns, and masks without government interference, media influence, and social media scolding. Once again I found out that I wasn't alone.

Initially I looked online to find other doctors supportive of hydroxychloroquine. There were dozens, even hundreds, who shared my conviction that the drug was a safe and effective treatment for COVID patients. Then I found others with stories to tell. Emails and calls went back and forth. Suddenly these experienced physicians were finding an outlet for their frustration. The community of medical professionals soon to be known as America's Frontline Doctors was taking shape. The days and weeks of bureaucratic frustration and clashes with my hospital's medical director receded into the past.

In early July, I traveled with five doctor colleagues to Washington, D.C. We met with Representatives Biggs, Perry, Norman, Bishop, Griffith, Doctors Caucus member Andy Harris, and other members of Congress as well as with an assistant to White House Chief of Staff Mark Meadows and an aide to Vice President Mike Pence. We expressed our concerns that the lockdowns were more damaging than the virus itself. Masking requirements were causing needless social divisiveness in a country already on edge.

We also discussed HCQ. A simple way to de-politicize the talk about HCQ was to make this effective generic drug available over the counter to all Americans who wanted it, we said. COVID wasn't smallpox. People could be trusted to balance risks and take precautions. Americans had come to know hydroxychloroquine—an uncontroversial drug—as an untried, even harmful, substance dispensed by quacks and eccentrics. Once the media pounced on President Trump's admission that he was taking the drug as a preventive measure on May 18, matters had only been made worse for patients and physicians across the country.

State health officials were already facing scrutiny related to thousands of nursing home deaths directly tied to their protocols for handling COVID-hospitalized patients. In May, 2.1 million Americans lived in nursing homes and assisted living facilities, representing 0.62 percent of the overall population but accounting for a staggering 42 percent of all COVID-19 deaths nationwide, according to the Foundation for Research on Equal Opportunity. They were now making another significant mistake that would increase suffering on a mass scale. Our leaders needed the political will to act. The virus would only defeat us if we defeated ourselves.

Even as I received more media exposure, I never promoted my views at work nor advocated for policy positions. Experience has taught me circumspection. I was well aware of doctors who had been targeted and threatened with termination, just for prescribing HCQ as a preventative or short-term treatment. There was Dr. Richard Urso, an ophthalmologist with a practice in Houston, Texas, who had worked with HCQ for thirty years but only received pushback from his state medical board in the COVID era. I knew Dr. Lionel Lee, a board-certified emergency medicine physician, ordered by his hospital to stop prescribing HCQ or face dismissal. A doctor from a southern state who asked not to be named was forced to not treat his very ill nursing home patients. Dr. Richard Price of Hawaii, Dr. Scott Campbell of Texas, and Dr. Richard Dubocq of Maine were all ordered by governors of their states not to prescribe a common generic medication. Still, I never thought it would happen to me.

America's Frontline Doctors returned to D.C. in late July. By this time our group had a website and a growing list of members. More importantly, we had support from thousands of everyday Americans tired of irrational and contradictory decrees from their cities and states. They believed there were other ways to manage this threat, and they were right.

Three AFLDS members who joined us around this time were Drs. James Todaro, Robert Hamilton, and Stella Immanuel.

Dr. Todaro is a trained ophthalmologist who earned his medical degree at Columbia University. Like me, Todaro is a free speech advocate; also like me, he's been targeted and persecuted by Big Tech and media for his views. Along with a partner, he published an important publicly available paper outlining the evidence for HCQ treatment. Todaro developed the first detailed exposé on the discredited *Lancet* study, "A Study Out of Thin Air." He would go on to serve as an Investigative Physician in AFLDS.

Dr. Hamilton was a general pediatrician in Santa Monica, California, for thirty-six years as well as the former President of the Los Angeles Pediatric Society. He studied medicine at UCLA Medical School, where he did his pediatric residency and chief residency. He's traveled to Africa on medical teams twenty-six times. His most recent trip was to Colombia to aid Venezuelan refugees leaving their country. Owing to his background in pediatrics, Dr. Hamilton is also the creator of a technique for calming crying babies that has been seen by over forty-four million viewers worldwide on YouTube.

Dr. Immanuel is a Cameroonian-American physician operating two clinics in Houston, Texas: a pediatric clinic and a general practice clinic. She practiced general medicine in Nigeria before immigrating to America to complete her residency as a pediatrician. By her own count, Dr. Immanuel treated more than five hundred patients successfully with HCQ.

I had planned the America's Frontline Doctors White Coat Summit for July 27. We hoped to educate the public and grow our network of physicians. We wanted to work with federal and state governments to make HCQ available to the public and advocate for best healthcare practices, including reopening schools and workplaces. We intended to fight on behalf of physicians who had been reprimanded or fired for prescribing HCQ, protect the doctor-patient relationship, and provide timely and actionable information to ordinary people based on the best available scientific and medical evidence.

The seven-hour AFLDS education summit featured around eighteen of us. The in-person event was held at a local nonprofit. My vision was to put doctors and social media influencers together in order to raise awareness and combat the massive amount of disinformation being generated by mainstream news organizations.

Although there were millions of views of the streaming educational sessions, they ended up being overshadowed by the press conference we conducted during a break between the morning and afternoon sessions on the steps of the U.S. Supreme Court. I picked the location because the High Court seemed like a natural choice. We were in a legal war over the rights of physicians, patients, and everyday Americans. I expected the Supreme Court one day to be the future venue of this medical-legal issue so I thought "Why not start there?" Chances are that's how you first learned about our group after the video went viral on news and social media sites.

"There are many thousands of physicians who have been silenced for telling the American people the good news about the situation, that we can manage the virus carefully and intelligently, but we cannot live with this spider web of fear that's constricting our country," I said at the Supreme Court. Dr. Hamilton talked about the sensitive issue of children attending school again. "We need to normalize the lives of our children. How do we do that? We do that by getting them back in the classroom. And the good news is they're not driving this infection at all. Yes, we can use security measures. Yes, we can be careful. I'm all for that. We all are. But I think the important thing is we need to not act out of fear," he said.

Here were doctors, many of them distinguished in their fields, talking directly to the American public—a public, I reasoned, as sick as I was of the Big Tech censorship, shifting government positions, and disinformation from both the medical establishment and media.

Our press conference garnered more than twenty million views on Facebook in about six hours. President Trump shared the video multiple times with his more than eighty-four million Twitter followers. Other influencers did the same.

I was totally unprepared for what would happen next.

"We've removed this video for sharing false information about cures and treatments for COVID-19," Facebook said through a curt and dismissive spokesperson that night.

We'd been censored and our video erased, purged from the collective digital memory in just a few hours.

Twitter censored the video in similar fashion. YouTube took down our video, too. So did Instagram. I couldn't help but remember what YouTube moderators did in April, when they removed a video of two California doctors who called for easing lockdown orders.

Now America's Frontline Doctors was being silenced as well.

The next day, still reeling, I was contacted by one of the hospitals where I worked. At the time, I had been working in the emergency departments of two hospitals. Hospital One was the site of my run-in with the medical director. Hospital Two was a low-income Native American hospital.

I was particularly proud of my emergency work there as such sites typically cannot attract board-certified emergency physicians. According to my superiors at Hospital Two, I had appeared in an "embarrassing video" and I could no longer work there.

In Washington I was speaking factually about my clinical experience caring for E.R. patients. I discussed facts and science, just not the ones that fit the media, government, or medical establishment's narrative at the time.

To my shock, I had been fired out of hand. Not only did Hospital Two refuse to put me on administrative leave, they threatened that if I did not go quietly they would pull the contract of the entire medical group that staffed its emergency department, with which I was affiliated. It's bad enough that I was terminated for speaking about my medical knowledge and experience. Here was an employer threatening my friends and colleagues for my free speech.

Not long after this I learned that the website-hosting company Squarespace had taken down the America's Frontline Doctors platform. Visitors to the website were met with an error message that the two-week-old website prepaid for one year had "expired."

I was still in Washington, trying to make sense of the previous day's events, and suddenly finding myself jobless and thousands of miles from home. What was I going to do? I had been a board-certified emergency physician for twenty years. It didn't seem so long ago that Americans of all backgrounds were (literally) cheering on people like me. I was a single working mother persecuted for talking honestly about my experience.

Shortly after speaking at the White Coat Summit, my AFLDS colleague Dr. Immanuel was threatened by the Texas Medical Board, the licensing authority in her state. She announced in August that she was being investigated by the board. Dr. Hamilton, who addressed legitimate concerns about deaths of despair in young people resulting from the lockdowns, a position supported by the American Academy of Pediatrics, was similarly vilified by the media and people in his community. Dr. Todaro, who had previously been censored by Google when the technology giant pulled down his HCQ white paper on March 23, continued to have his work flagged or suppressed.

I was overwhelmed and shocked. It was like being caught in a whirlwind. I was upset and scared that I was fired. At the same time, I was being invited to give interviews and share my story with the likes of Tucker Carlson, Glenn Beck, Dennis Prager, and KUSI News. The experience was surreal. I had a Twitter account, but I didn't start using it until April. By June it had grown to about two thousand followers. The week of the summit the number exploded to over one hundred thousand. People were reaching out with messages of gratitude while the media relentlessly tried to discredit our cause. Each day was an emotional seesaw.

I never anticipated that these actions would jeopardize my medical career. AFLDS members had volunteered to come to Washington, D.C. All these physicians paid their own way and volunteered hours and days of their time. This wasn't about money or fame. Experts here and abroad had produced a compendium of sources demonstrating that HCQ was safe and effective for treating COVID-19. We had the facts on our side. Yet the vicious media attacks rained down. *HuffPost* called us "quacks." Vice saved their ire for Trump and others sharing what they described as "lies and misinformation." A reporter for the CBS affiliate in Los Angeles took to social media to declare that none of us were "actually frontline doctors." And on and on.

My intention had been to raise awareness about an overlooked and effective treatment, but medical cancel culture had other ideas. (It was highly ironic that one of our educational sessions was on medical cancel culture.)

These critics hadn't walked in my shoes. They hadn't treated patients at 2 a.m. after spending a whole day in an emergency department. They weren't there to witness the recovery of Patient One, just as the medical literature had indicated. I was defamed by the media, censored by social media companies, terminated by my employers, and viciously attacked, all for advocating for the right of physicians to do what they always had done in America: prescribe what they believe is best for their patients. If it can happen to me, it can happen to anyone.

At the time of the AFLDS summit, I said that fear of the virus was draining the lifeblood of the American people, American society, and the American economy. I learned that this fear has had three major effects.

First, "the news" became less about providing actionable and timely information for the public and more about telling us what to think according to their political prerogatives. Second, HCQ, a significant factor in the medical debate, was marginalized in public conversation to the detriment of millions of patients. There is also an unhealthy obsession in the media with Donald Trump. Because he endorsed HCQ, the treatment was dismissed out of hand. Yet the science is clearly there to support its use in treating COVID-19.

Third, what was emerging in hospitals like mine was something like a medical-sickness-trauma complex, amplified by the media and taking its cues from voices high in the federal bureaucracy. It made the normal practice of medicine an offense against the state. Take Dr. Fauci's blatantly unscientific statements during an interview on MSN-BC on July 29: "On trials that are valid, that were randomized and controlled in the proper way, all of those trials show consistently that hydroxychloroquine is not effective in the treatment of coronavirus disease or COVID-19." The comments came a day after President Trump reiterated his support for the drug.

Meanwhile, millions of unused HCQ doses sat in the Strategic National Stockpile. The American College of Emergency Physicians and the American Academy of Emergency Medicine lined up behind Fauci shortly thereafter. I didn't blame the president for keeping Dr. Fauci on the Coronavirus Task Force. After all, the NIAID director was popular and President Trump had other battles to focus on without starting a fresh media dust-up. Given these circumstances I would've acted similarly. Still, Fauci has repeatedly contradicted himself and has been consistently inaccurate on a massive scale, and I welcomed President Trump adding new members with different perspectives to the Task Force, which ultimately he did.

I've witnessed much negative change to the practice of medicine over the course of my life—first as the daughter of a doctor and then during my own career. Our experience with infectious diseases, from SARS in 2002 followed later by the Ebola scare in 2014, or dramatic technological advances like robotic surgery, have not contributed much to those changes. The real problem is the gradual intrusion of big government into the doctor-patient relationship, adding impossible and conflicting paperwork, red tape, and insoluble obstructions without improving the quality of care for the people I meet in hospital emergency rooms.

This trend was already established. But when it came to the coronavirus pandemic, something radically different was taking place. Big Tech and Big Media cancel culture were new obstacles to patient care.

I have never considered myself a political person. I've supported both parties at various times in my life. I'd fall in the middle of any partisan test. I don't believe in the right-left distinction. I believe in the Constitution and in what I do as a doctor to help people live better lives. That's the trouble with being in the middle of the road. Sometimes you get run over. I was determined not to let these setbacks deter me, however. I might have lost my job and been muzzled by Big Tech's digital commissars, but I would continue to speak my mind and let other independent-minded Americans decide for themselves.

III.

WHAT THE SCIENCE SAYS: THE TRUTH ABOUT HCQ

How did it happen that an ordinary, widely used antimalarial drug that shares a chemical blueprint with the quinine found in tree bark, became the target of a coordinated campaign of misinformation and deception? All of a sudden hydroxychloroquine was not the safe and effective treatment I along with thousands of other doctors had prescribed to patients countless times without controversy. It certainly wasn't the medicine derived from the South American cinchona tree that Gen. George Washington administered to the Continental Army as a malaria preventative and that has been widely used **for centuries.**

Now HCQ was public enemy number one, an allegedly "obscure drug" offering "false hope" to Americans young and old, in the phrasing of typical mainstream news articles.

My first professional obligation is to the patient. In the case of COVID-19, the well-being of my patients depended on their timely access to accurate information about potentially life-saving treatments. That information was outright censored in the national drama that was unfolding after President Trump uttered the words "hydroxychloroquine" and "game changer" together on March 19.

Science, once the disinterested handmaiden of medicine grounded in evidence and experimentation, now became just another target in the culture war. Increasing government intrusion made patient-centered healthcare almost impossible in this environment. And most tragic of all, the aggressive campaign against HCQ cost half to three-quarters of the two hundred thousand American lives attributed to COVID-19.

By their own admission, leading medical journals printed anti-HCQ junk science masquerading as research. Having the temerity to call this out, as some of us did, meant courting both professional ridicule and vicious media attacks. Even worse was Big Tech's censorship and online cancel culture via the digital mob.

Despite all this, physicians have an imperative to live within the truth. The Hippocratic Oath, not political correctness nor government decree, must determine our actions as doctors.

It wasn't until late January 2020 that the Chinese government admitted to human-to-human transmission of a new coronavirus, named corona for the "crown" of spiky proteins the virus appears to wear when viewed under a microscope. At the time, I had already started reading the medical literature about the respiratory illness from Wuhan, China, that ultimately became known as COVID-19.

SARS-CoV-2 was the third respiratory virus that had escaped from China in the past twenty-five years: first the bird flu in 1996, then the original SARS in 2002, then 2013's H7N9. COVID-19 was the seventh confirmed human coronavirus, a lineage that includes the common cold as well as lethal viruses like Middle East respiratory syndrome, known as MERS.

Soon after registering California's first case, our hospitals were being briefed on new protocols related to treating COVID-19. A hospital tent had been set up. There were updated hospitalization procedures enacted to protect non-COVID patients. The discussions were extensive but necessary. Daily and even hourly conversations ensued. But there was one topic that wasn't addressed: the use of hydroxychloroquine.

For all the attention paid to this medication since, in hindsight it's illuminating to consider HCQ's near-total absence from our early, often freewheeling talks on how to respond to this threat. It just wasn't brought up one way or the other in any critical manner. There was certainly no mention of reprimands if doctors used their professional judgment to dispense it. We sometimes mentioned HCQ mildly, amiably, much like thousands of similar conversations I have had over the years with colleagues about treatments. Some thought it sounded promising; others thought it didn't; most didn't care at all. But, certainly, no one ever suggested it was dangerous. That was January and February and March.

When things changed, I was joined by my colleagues in America's Frontline Doctors to set the record straight on hydroxychloroquine and empower patients to seek out this safe, effective, common, and cost-effective prescription drug as both a curative and preventive treatment against COVID-19. The foundation for my educational effort was a white paper I authored in July 2020 making the case for HCQ using current scientific and historical data. Unlike the powerful interests intent on silencing me and removing HCQ from hospitals and pharmacies, I was actually going to follow the science and let patients make up their own minds based on the best available evidence. After all, neither political agendas nor media influence should drive these critical decisions for doctors and patients. When those forces shape a medical discussion, the consequences are always dire.

As a doctor I know there are only two things to be considered regarding a medication: Is it safe and does it work? Hydroxychloroquine was approved as a medical treatment by the Food and Drug Administration over sixty-five years ago. Since that time, it has been used by more than two billion—yes, billion with a "B"—patients worldwide. HCQ is sold over the counter (OTC) to people in most of Latin America, Africa, and Southeast Asia but it is available only by prescription in the United States. To be clear, this is not because the drug is unsafe for Americans to use without consulting a doctor. In fact, it's typically sold in the vitamin section of stores across the world. The reason it is only sold by prescription in the United States has to do with our domestic pharmaceutical processes. No one from Big Pharma has ever requested that hydroxychloroquine be sold over the counter. My allies and I in AFLDS want to see this changed.

A prescription drug can become an over-the-counter drug if a pharmaceutical manufacturer petitions the FDA to update its status. There are scores of medications that were previously available by prescription-only, among them Aleve, Motrin, Zantac, Pepcid, Antivert, Benadryl, Claritin, Rogaine—even nicotine gum.

HCQ manufacturers haven't brought an OTC petition to the FDA because consumer over-the-counter demand for the drug here is almost nonexistent. It's also cheap. Countries such as France, whose citizens travel more often to malaria-prone regions, previously did stock HCQ on their shelves. In America, where hydroxychloroquine is primarily used to treat conditions like rheumatoid arthritis and lupus, it is much less often used as a preventative and treatment for malaria.

It is therefore manifestly a lack of profit potential, not safety concerns, that's kept HCQ off American drug store shelves. Up until March 2020, there was no consumer demand for over-the-counter HCQ in America. Now, as more people learn about the benefits of treatment with hydroxychloroquine, I hope consumer demand will inspire pharmaceutical companies to seek FDA approval for over-the-counter status of the drug.

It so happens that each of these illnesses—rheumatoid arthritis, lupus, and malaria—involves a distinct patient category. It's why HCQ has been used for decades in all types of people: from children to pregnant women, breastfeeding women, young and healthy travelers, to the elderly and the immunocompromised. The drug is safe. We know this because it's been taken by vastly different people in a variety of settings over the years.

Media clickbait routinely calls HCQ dangerous and points to its supposed ties to cardiac issues. Yet in my research, I found that in the largest study to date on the topic, HCQ has been shown not to increase heart risk. This paper was authored by scientists from thirty-three countries and companies across the world. It studied all the data from the years 2000 through 2020 on patients who were prescribed HCQ. The study had two goals: first, to understand the safety of HCQ by itself as a monotherapy; second, to record its safety when paired with the antibiotic azithromycin.

The study, "Safety of hydroxychloroquine, alone and in combination with azithromycin, in light of rapid widespread use for COVID-19: a multinational, network cohort and self-controlled case series study," found that over a twenty-year period, looking at almost one million patients, those taking HCQ did not have an increased risk of heart problems. According to the study's authors: "This is the largest-ever analysis of the safety of such treatments worldwide, examining over 900,000 HCQ and more than 300,000 HCQ + azithromycin users respectively. The results on the risk of serious adverse events associated with short-term (one month) HCQ treatment as proposed for COVID-19 therapy are reassuring, with no excess risk of any of the considered safety outcomes compared to an equivalent therapy."

The Food and Drug Administration's database shows a total of only 640 deaths attributable to HCQ over fifty years. To put this in context, 640 deaths represents 0.034 percent of all the deaths (1,910,212) attributable to medications over the same period. Compare this infinitesimal number to the 458 deaths caused by over-the-counter Tylenol in 2019 in the US alone. The FDA goes on to say, "Each year the FDA receives over 1 million adverse event reports associated with the use of drug products. This concerns the entirety of HCQ use over more than 50 years of data, likely millions of uses and of longer-term use than the five days recommended for COVID-19 treatment."

Far from an outlier in the federal bureaucracy, the FDA's opinion on hydroxychloroquine's safety is echoed by CDC scientists. For example, the agency prepared an information sheet about HCQ for people who have questions regarding malaria prevention and treatment. That sheet includes the following: "Hydroxychloroquine can be prescribed to adults and children of all ages. It can also be safely taken by pregnant women and nursing mothers."

About treatment length and potential side effects, the question-and-answer guide states, "Hydroxychloroquine is a relatively well tolerated medicine. The most common adverse reactions reported are stomach pain, nausea, vomiting, and headache. CDC has no limits on the use of hydroxychloroquine for the prevention of malaria."

It is well established that there is no scientific basis for the claim that HCQ is risky on its own. The only credible theory as to why there has even been a concern is that since the beginning, possible treatment options of COVID-19 have always included HCQ in combination with the antibiotic azithromycin. Taken together, it has been alleged by publications like *The American Journal of Managed Care* that there could be a serious and frequent enough concern that people should not use HCQ for COVID-19. But the American Heart Association has now rendered a verdict on this specific question. They found that taking HCQ, even in combination with azithromycin, does not cause an increased risk of fatal heart-rhythm problems, in particular "no instances of Torsade de pointes, or arrhythmogenic death were reported."

In addition, for years HCQ has been listed on the World Health Organization's (WHO) Model List of Essential

Medicines, remedies known as "the most efficacious, safe and cost-effective medicines for priority conditions." My own research revealed that more than five hundred million tablets of hydroxychloroquine are dispensed in the United States every year. Unlike many drugs, hydroxychloroquine is also not addictive. Finally, this time-tested and commonly prescribed therapeutic is also low-cost. The total treatment cost for COVID-19 is around **ten dollars.**

It was critically important to me to tell Americans that the CDC, FDA, American Heart Association, and even the WHO all regarded hydroxychloroquine as safe. The media blackout at first stymied my efforts, but I wouldn't be deterred. This was our primary task after I formed America's Frontline Doctors. We aggressively, emphatically, explicitly, unmistakably, unambiguously said that hydroxychloroquine is safe. There is no data, absolutely none, to indicate that HCQ should be withheld from the American people, we repeated despite the **media attacks.**

We know that if the media, politicians, and scientists won't acknowledge the irrefutable evidence that this medication is safe, they certainly won't be honest about its effectiveness, which is a newer and more nuanced issue. However, America's Frontline Doctors main message is one of hope: the evidence for HCQ's effectiveness against COVID-19 is **overwhelming.**

Viruses spend virtually all of their time and energy replicating themselves inside a host cell. In fact, the singular goal of a virus is to make more viruses. A drug that interferes with a virus's ability to replicate itself will neutralize it. Chemically speaking, HCQ acts as the doorman to the cell, allowing zinc to march in behind it, and it is actually the zinc which halts the viral reproduction. Zinc jams the genetic photocopier, to be sure, but HCQ enables zinc to get inside the cell in the first place.

CDC researchers further attested to CQ's effectiveness as a therapeutic and prophylactic against SARS coronavirus when they described how it raises the cell's pH levels. In doing so the drug inhibits the ability of the virus to fuse with and attack cells. According to one study using primate cells, the drug successfully reduced infection and spread even after infection. CDC's study goes on to note "the infectivity of coronaviruses other than SARS-CoV are also affected by chloroquine."

There was a similar pandemic to COVID-19 over fifteen years ago. The two illnesses are so similar in fact that they share a name. It turns out the "novel" coronavirus known as COVID-19 is not so novel after all. SARS-CoV-1 (from China in 2002) and SARS-CoV-2 (from China in 2019) are 78 percent identical.

At the beginning of the SARS-CoV-1 outbreak, physicians started to treat that respiratory disease with chloroquine (CQ). In subsequent patient guidelines, Chinese research scientists concluded: "Expert consensus on chloroquine phosphate for new coronavirus pneumonia: ... clinical research results show that chloroquine improves the success rate of treatment and shortens the length of patient's hospital stay." Similarly positive guidelines emerged from South Korea's Biomedical Review. What unites these two countries in their opinion of HCQ? Experience. Time and exposure to a highly infectious respiratory condition such as SARS-CoV-1, a close relative of today's novel coronavirus, illustrated the effectiveness of antimalarial therapies. The findings in East Asia were so persuasive that Virology, a peer-reviewed journal established in 1955, published this headline back in 2005: "Chloroquine is a potent inhibitor of SARS coronavirus infection and spread."

Around the start of the current pandemic, one of the most renowned microbiologists specializing in infectious diseases in the world was the aforementioned Dr. Didier Raoult, an acclaimed scientist who wanted to demonstrate that HCQ could be used to save patients from COVID-19, exactly as chloroquine had slowed reproduction of the SARS coronavirus in cell cultures back in 2002. Brilliant yet contrarian, Dr. Raoult has been the recipient of the Grand Prix Inserm, one of France's top scientific prizes. Dr. Raoult had already suggested in a 2007 research paper that chloroquine and hydroxychloroquine might be "an interesting weapon to face present and future infectious diseases worldwide."

With COVID-19, he now had his chance to test this theory in the field. Dr. Raoult first published his own study of a group of thirty-six patient participants at his medical clinic in Marseilles; sixteen were in the control group. After less than a week, all six COVID-19 patients treated with a combination of HCQ and azithromycin tested negative for the virus. Raoult published his findings on March 4 as "Chloroquine and hydroxychloroquine as available weapons to fight COVID-19" in the International Journal of Antimicrobial Agents.

The evidence for HCQ's effectiveness is piling up fast and furious. As AFLDS explained in July 2020, "When examining data on efficacy, Dr. Risch notes that evidence against HCQ when it is used alone is irrelevant, as it has been known since Feb-March that HCQ must be used in combination therapy." So much for the safety and efficacy "concerns" trotted out by corrupt scientific journals and amplified by an agenda and hysteria-driven media establishment. At the time of this writing, there are more than eighty studies from around the world proving HCQ is effective against COVID-19. This includes studies conducted in China, France, South Korea, New York state, India, Brazil, Iran, Saudi Arabia, Mexico, Portugal, Detroit, New York City, Belgium, and more.

A starkly positive study looking at combination HCQ and AZM therapies for hospitalized patients in the Detroit area published in the *International Journal of Infectious Diseases* found "In this multi-hospital assessment, when controlling for COVID-19 risk factors, treatment with HCQ alone and in combination with AZM was associated with reduction in COVID-19 mortality," cutting mortality rates in half. The Detroit study was completed in early May but its publication was delayed until the Friday before the July Fourth holiday, effectively hiding it from a public who no doubt would have welcomed the findings as further proof of HCQ's usefulness. Whether this delay was collusion between the scientific-medical establishment and the media is hard to say. Nonetheless, valuable time in the fight against COVID-19 was lost.

Hydroxychloroquine is safe, effective, and should be made available over the counter to Americans just as it is in most of Africa, South America, much of Asia, and even Iran. Unfortunately, powerful forces are holding it back in first-world democracies such as the United States, United Kingdom, the Netherlands, Belgium, France, Ireland, Sweden, and Canada. What has the spiral into anti-scientific hysteria cost our society?

If Dr. Fauci believes that "science is truth," as he has said, then large segments of the world's medical, political, and media elite have been living a lie since January, when French authorities incredibly demoted HCQ from an over-the-counter drug to "poisonous substance" and Canada quietly removed it from pharmacy shelves. As I wrote in the AFLDS white paper, "Given that CQ was demonstrated to be very effective against a 78 percent identical coronavirus less than 15 years ago during a very similar situation, it is very curious that there was a multinational effort to restrict it starting in mid-January."

Could more lives have been saved from this potentially lethal disease with over-the-counter HCQ? Absolutely. Again, Yale's Dr. Risch: "US cumulative deaths through

July 15 are 140,000. Had we permitted HCQ use liberally, we would have saved half, 70,000 and it is very possible we could have saved 3/4, 105,000." At the same time, we are just beginning to tally the fatal consequences COVID-19 has had for those not exposed to the virus. According to the CDC's National Center for Health Statistics, there were between 202,000 and 263,000 excess deaths through late August 2020.

The US by that point had 188,000 known deaths attributed to COVID-19, according to the Center for Health Security at Johns Hopkins University. Medical researchers from the Robert Wood Johnson Foundation found 20 percent non-COVID-related excess deaths between February 1 and late August. Stress, anxiety, and financial pressures could all contribute to the higher weekly deaths in 2020 attributable to fatal heart attacks, diabetes, strokes, and hypertension. This excess death due to non-COVID phenomena was predictable and was the subject of the letter that I wrote to the President in May, co-signed by seven hundred other physicians.

By ignoring recent history and credible scientific data, doctors and public health officials broke their Hippocratic Oath. However, I believe there is still time to evaluate the evidence and make HCQ accessible to any citizen who wants it as we continue to deal with this pandemic.

Inaction and confusing narratives are making Americans more anxious about their well-being, forcing them to put off necessary medical care, locking them down inside a prison of fear. Once Americans know they can buy a safe, cheap, generic, life-saving medication should they need it—or as a preventive measure—the normal patterns of life can be restored. For example, a person who suffers from an occasional migraine headache but who has the migraine medicine at home or in her pocket, in case she needs it, is a person who feels safe and comfortable going about her daily routine. If she does not have that prescription, she may limit herself a lot or a little, and either way, she is fearful of what could be right around the corner.

If this state of affairs continues, patients and their families will lose. Medical science will lose, too. Understandably, people have become suspicious of science. The victors in this game will be Big Pharma and corporate giants that can continue to make money off pricey treatments. The winners will be those in our politics, Big Media, and Big Tech who stoke fear for financial or political gain.

I consider myself fortunate to practice medicine and to use my skills to help others. Like so many other physicians, I got into medicine to save lives, to reduce suffering, and help people live better. Medicine is a noble profession, although it has changed dramatically over the years and decades. Much of it hasn't been for the better in terms of patient care. The corruption in our system destroys lives and spreads suffering. We can stop it with the truth.

IV.

WHY DID THIS HAPPEN—AND WHAT CAN WE DO?

When asked what inner support I fall back on in difficult times, like many Americans I'll include my religious faith on that list. I don't consider myself a devout person. In my opinion, few of us are truly strong enough to make that journey. We often fall short of the ideal God sets before us. Instead, I seek the glimpses of transcendent truth only religion can provide. When I share a Shabbat meal with family or friends, I'm continuing an ancient ritual that sets aside time and place to bear witness to God's truth, outside the messy realm of human affairs. Rabbi Abraham Heschel called the observance of the Jewish sabbath, the day of rest, "A palace in time in which we build." From our journey up the mountain of life we pause to look out and attempt to perceive the meaning of His plan for us, if only partially.

Months into the pandemic and we were still asking for truth. Months of hysteria had left Americans scared and more polarized than ever before. We were flying for each other's throats over minor transgressions. We were talking about raw case numbers and masks instead of much more important indicators like mortality, positivity, hospitalizations, or even recoveries.

Healthcare often isn't about treating people. Powerful interests including insurance carriers, drug companies, the federal government, and an activist news media have distorted the picture of medicine beyond recognition. The goal of these interests isn't to seek scientific truth, or even to keep us healthy. As a result, the physician's profession is changing in dramatic and troubling ways.

A conscious effort on the part of the media and many politicians was to drive fear instead of hope. Ordinary people have suffered enormous economic hardship and mental distress whose effects may echo down to future generations. America's largest cities were locked down for months, destroying businesses and draining the life savings of millions. Americans faced deep financial hardship through no fault of their own. Jobless claims topped one million week after week as businesses shut their doors. The US hit an all-time high of more than 6.2 million weekly claims in early April. Schoolchildren suffered academic and social losses for the sake of driving a narrative and an active effort to keep the truth from people.

There was no scientific justification for the consistent hostility to HCQ, so what was the explanation? Why did this happen? My experiences as an emergency doctor and later as a public health advocate for ordinary Americans who desperately want to get back to a normal life have provided me with a few clues.

Cui bono: "who benefits?" A simple Latin phrase every law student encounters. After the censoring of the AFLDS video, the deep-sixing of our website, and the defamatory stories in the mainstream press, "cui bono" stuck in my head. The lawyer in me analyzed the problem, diligently. I kept turning over its legal implications like paging through volumes of cases. The doctor in me returned to the Hippocratic Oath, the basis of medical ethics. What was driving these various sources of influence and power—medicine, government, technology, and media—to limit the public's access to a safe and effective generic drug sold like vitamins in countries outside the United States?

I came to view it as a nexus of the malign effects of politicized science, the profit motive, and the politics of fear.

As resistance grew to my prescribing HCQ and irrational behavior from administrative staff and my colleagues increased, I started to better understand our divergent worldviews. The bumper-sticker directive to "follow the science" was actually an evasion of responsibility. It lets people off the hook for their bad decisions in a crisis. Was New York Governor Cuomo's executive order sending COVID-hospitalized patients back to nursing homes to infect other vulnerable nursing home patients "following the science"? Of course not. And sending post-hospitalization COVID-positive patients back to nursing homes was unnecessary. Relative to the total nursing home population, Governor Cuomo contributed to a larger percentage of nursing-home deaths—especially when compared to the states without such a policy. New Jersey's over seven thousand nursing home deaths account for half of the state's fatalities since March. Pennsylvania did just as miserably. These governors made specific decisions that cost thousands of the most vulnerable their lives. But they didn't do it to their own relatives.

As reported by local and national media including Newsweek, Dr. Rachel Levine, Pennsylvania's secretary of health, moved her ninety-five-year-old mother out of an assisted living facility at the exact same time Pennsylvania ordered nursing homes to accept COVID-positive patients. Science was being perverted into spin and cheap ways to stage-manage bad public policy. It is shameful.

Science isn't absolute. It can be wrong. There are always disagreements and dissent. The discipline also isn't an article of faith. Its credibility depends on flesh-and-blood human beings testing generalized theories against new evidence. But human beings can fall short, and science can become politicized right under our noses. The American Medical Association (AMA) is the modern-day embodiment of politicized science. The AMA has been captured by political interests since at least 2009. Instead of advocating for physician discretion and patient care, the nation's largest medical organization lined up against HCQ and ordinary practitioners trying to save lives. When it came down to the basic facts of HCQ, our overconfident and worldly-wise so-called scientific "experts" turned out to understand little about their own profession.

Fear paralyzed too many in the scientific-medical establishment. Fear of ridicule scared off early dissenters from the need for lockdowns and alternative approaches to treatment. Then fear of professional sanction—medical cancel culture—amplified by the mainstream media, kept them afraid. Political thinkers in Machiavelli's time and likely before understood that fear is more important than love or respect to a ruling elite. Divided by fear, citizens are easier to control. Before we knew it, Americans were captured by this spreading spider web: paralyzed, isolated, and vulnerable to multiple threats.

Taken in this light, our AFLDS summit and its fallout was eye-opening. Reading reporters' tweets about our supposed lack of credentials or listening to cable news anchors getting the science wrong was like sitting in on the meeting of a political opposition research team. The first step, in their view, was misinformation (HCQ isn't effective; failure to report the positive studies). Then, disinformation

Simone Gold, M.D., J.D.

(HCQ isn't safe; report the negative studies and ignore later retractions). Finally, when the previous two don't work, full-on censorship. We were quite possibly watching free speech in its death throes, I told one interviewer recently. Fear is now affecting something as basic as physical health.

Big Media and Big Tech have manipulated the social reality of America and of Americans. At some point it becomes almost impossible to change minds quickly enough to save lives. The Faustian bargain Americans made with technology companies has been laid bare in the COVID crisis. The platform gatekeepers of digital media expanded the diffusion of certain information—some helpful but some not—while raising the chances that other knowledge could be hidden from the public without explanation.

Big Tech's history of erasing content on its platforms at odds with the wisdom of so-called experts or a specific agenda is directly in conflict with our nation's history of fostering free speech and threatens the civic life of a democratic republic. Look at Google's behavior in the case of my AFLDS colleague Dr. James Todaro's HCQ white paper. The tech company banned the document on March 23, in the early days of the pandemic, without warning to Dr. Todaro or his co-author Gregory Rigano. No explanation from Google was forthcoming either. Users were simply brought to an empty page. Twitter placed warnings on tweets linking to the phantom document. Was this action consistent with "Don't be evil," Google's much-cited code of conduct? Their opposition to HCQ had nothing to do with codes of conduct, or science for that matter. The best meme from this time was a picture of a young girl holding a sign which read "If only child pornography was taken down from social media as fast as information about hydroxychloroquine."

Compound this with the actions of big government and Big Pharma. Profit-seeking elements within society had plenty of reasons to keep private access to HCQ limited to a doctor's prescription and subject to the control of state pharmacy boards and public authorities. Other Big Pharma drugs for on-label use needed to move to the front of the line. At ten dollars for the entire treatment, HCQ simply didn't qualify as a money-maker. Its favorable position as a common generic, therefore, was standing between the drug companies and more-profitable products to sell the American public. Treatments such as vaccines cannot jump ahead for one of the FDA's emergency use authorizations if there is an on-label therapeutic such as HCQ in front of it. Simply put, Big Pharma did not stand to make enough money from existing medications. Something had to give. That something was patient care.

Parts of the state and federal governments abused their power and the trust the public had placed in them. It shouldn't matter whether the president is a Republican or Democrat. It shouldn't matter whether they are popular or not. Public health is supposed to be non-partisan. When a crisis hits, manipulating science to serve a political agenda is fundamentally dangerous. It costs lives. We learned this the hard way with hydroxychloroquine. A government powerful enough to control your physician or your hospital has proven it can limit your treatment choices to your detriment.

In the end, the pharmaceutical industry, government, and the scientific-medical establishment shoved HCQ aside to make room for more expensive, and therefore more profitable, treatments. That would be Gilead's antiviral medication remdesivir, which can cost over $4,000, but even more incentivized are the pharmaceutical manufacturers of vaccines. In this way, vaccines treat the pre-infected and remdesivir manages the disease in its late stages, such as those already hospitalized. In the case of France, the naked profit motive was there in January 2020, well before the virus had a global foothold. To this day, I know of no other instance in which public health officials reverted an over-the-counter drug back to prescription, as the French did at the start of 2020. Just as in the United States, HCQ's reputation in France was tried, tested, and true.

When the cozy relationship among science, government, and business filtered down to the state level, the results for the average citizen weren't pretty. Much like in war, the first casualty of this alliance was the ability for frontline doctors like me to speak the truth. Through power and fear, state government officials chilled discussion from alternative voices and created an echo chamber of politically correct opinions. State governors like Gavin Newsom of California have taken outsized roles in personal medical decisions. They've turned pharmacists into regulatory arms of the state.

The last remaining inviolable corner of the universe is the doctor-patient relationship. Imagine as a physician being on the phone with a pharmacist and they refuse to fill a prescription. These aren't just anecdotes from cranky doctors. There are voluminous examples on YouTube and elsewhere online documenting the obstruction of physician independence and discretion because pharmacists are taking orders from their politically influenced state boards and corporate employers.

Telling doctors they can't use an off-label, FDA-approved drug to treat patients is an unprecedented power grab and in essence practicing medicine without a license, which is still illegal. Twenty-one percent of all prescriptions are "off-label," after all. It is a meaningless phrase to a physician.

If the Big Media-Big Tech censorship machine can be effective against such a safe, decades-old drug, they can make the American public believe anything. This is one of the reasons I am fighting so hard. From my perspective, it is as though they have all of America believing that Tylenol is dangerous, or grapefruits, or fruit punch. Corrupted science, fear, and profit-seeking are at the core of opposition to this beneficial drug for widespread use. They combined to get me fired as an emergency doctor and literally censored me. Mark Zuckerberg, in the halls of Congress, called what I said "disinformation." It is hard for me to imagine someone like my physician father practicing medicine today, with its politics, compromised "experts," and social media barons serving as mouthpieces for the medical community.

When I decided to speak out, I didn't intend to change the course of my whole life. After all, I love medicine. I liked being a doctor on the frontlines of healthcare. My patients' well-being came first. It was only when conditions changed that the decision to step out of my chosen profession and into the role of public health advocate occurred. Or perhaps it was an inevitability set in motion by unprecedented events.

Fear is like radioactivity: once released, it filters into everything. But we can stop being afraid by choosing to live joyfully in hope. The first president of post-communist Czechoslovakia, Vaclav Havel, said, "Hope is not the same thing as optimism. It is … the certainty that something makes sense, regardless of how it turns out." Hope is the lead shield protecting us from radioactive fear.

So how do we protect ourselves, our health, and those we love from this kind of interference? How do we collectively fight medical cancel culture?

Despite the power wielded by our unaccountable elites, ordinary Americans can take steps toward recovering their country by overcoming fear. Stop being afraid of everyday interactions due to COVID. Return to a healthy social life. Go out with friends or enjoy time with your family. If you're a religious person, renew your spiritual commitments by attending a local house of worship. Most importantly, be grateful that we still live in a free country where these rights are protected by our Constitution. Do these things while being mindful about your overall risk in all health issues.

When it comes to safely reopening schools, there is no evidence that in-person instruction poses an increased risk to students and there is enormous evidence of the increased risk to students' well-being from distance learning. Unfortunately, it has proven impossible to get leaders to act dispassionately. Innovative parents have responded to this government-induced chaos by creating private "micro-schools" of ten or fewer students each. Parents share supervisory duties for students who choose to learn remotely, or they pool resources to hire a private tutor to oversee the micro-school class, or both. What does not make sense is scaring parents and children over something that does not exist and disrupting kids' lives. Parents should refuse to participate in what is tantamount to government-sanctioned child abuse.

I'm not advocating for those with certain comorbidities such as obesity, hypertension, diabetes, or the elderly to throw caution to the wind. Your risk of a bad outcome infection increases if you are in one of these groups and you do not receive early treatment. However, understand what reasonable risk looks like and use your own judgment instead of having politicians or bureaucrats decide for you how to live your life. A life spent minimizing risk to the greatest possible degree will be a life wasted.

Not everyone can, or should, turn to political activism. I fully understand those who point out the negative consequences this approach can have for one's career and personal life. I get it. But people don't have to be public figures to learn to fortify themselves against misinformation and coercion. Going along with the crowd in times of fear and uncertainty present their own pitfalls, as we have seen. In Judaism we often ask ourselves, "What does God expect of me in this situation?" It's this emphasis on action that is essential to the Jewish faith. Trust in God, believe in yourself, and courageous conduct will follow.

We can return to normalcy by filtering out the media noise related to the virus. Clickbait journalism produces nothing but hair-raising headlines designed to keep us fixated on negativity. Sure, it makes them money, but it also harms you. With the worst of COVID-19 likely behind us, mainstream press outlets desperate for eyeballs cherry-pick statistics in an effort to paint the worst possible picture. These amateur epidemiologists endlessly talk about "seven-day rolling averages" and "highest single-day cases" while missing basic details that would get a first-year medical student bounced from her class.

Incremental and anecdotal infection cases are irrelevant. Total numbers are irrelevant. Most of these are not even "cases" but just positive test results. Most will experience no symptoms or mild to moderate symptoms and recover quickly. Many international studies show that countries that use HCQ as an early treatment for COVID patients have an exponentially lower mortality rate. You'll never hear that in the United States.

Do the research and decide for yourself.

It's also imperative that we repair the doctor-patient relationship damaged by intrusive government action. If you're seeking better treatment options for a possible coronavirus infection, make sure your physician has seen the data recommending HCQ as an early intervention.

One mom sent me a note after her twenty-five-year-old son contracted the virus: "My husband sent him a link to your site and told him to read the research. He did. He was convinced by the science that HCQ was safe, contacted a doctor, and received a prescription for HCQ within 24 hours. He felt much better the next day and is currently on the mend."

In my opinion, this is one of the most important priorities right now for the medical community and doctors who want to practice without unreasonable agenda-driven restrictions. We can't let experts far from the frontlines treat politicized science like religious tablets presented to the unenlightened.

I know that activism against medical cancel culture can work. It matters a lot to me that certain laws have changed after I and my colleagues took up the fight for access to effective COVID treatment. Six states have since relaxed their controls on HCQ. Within two weeks of our Summit, President Trump appointed the well-respected Dr. Scott Atlas to the White House Coronavirus Task Force. Dr.

Atlas has been among other things a top healthcare advisor to presidential candidates and now provides the president with an alternative view to Dr. Fauci's. People in the medical world believe my work had something to do with it. For a person like me, this is satisfying. Of course, Dr. Atlas has also become a victim of smear campaigns and outright censorship at the hands of the same cabal that came after me and America's Frontline Doctors.

We still have the freedom to choose. Understand your medical rights and seek out physicians who respect these rights. Self-appointed experts and their allies in the media can only rule us by fear as long as we remain afraid. It's time for Americans to live fearlessly again. How do we do this given a range of unknowns and a changing environment? A related question is one I am asked frequently and provides the reason for writing this book: "It was easy for you—you're a doctor and lawyer. But how can I know what the truth is?"

This haunts me more than any other question. COVID-19 has proven that the American people can be dangerously misled, to the tune of hundreds of thousands of deaths, more than 30 percent unemployment, and a stalled world economy. It has proven that the average American is worse off listening to the American media than listening to nothing. This disease has also proven that the disinformation campaign can be so complete as to negate our fundamental rights as human beings to live in the freedom guaranteed by our Constitution.

The evidence is overwhelming that the American people were lied to, but I can appreciate that the disinformation was not clear to the average person at the time. For this reason I developed a six-point strategy (and acronym) that concerned citizens must use to decide what to believe before the next disinformation campaign is unleashed.

First, don't spend any time wondering about anyone's motives. This is not a banal suggestion to assume the best about other people. Rather it is because your lack of imagination into other people's motives will cause you to disbelieve the facts. You must accept that on a fundamental level no one can ever be entirely certain of another's motives. Every single day I heard people say, "Well I don't believe that because, why would the CDC do that? Why would the FDA do that?" Just because the questioner cannot imagine motive does not mean the evidence isn't there. The way to avoid this type of faulty thinking is to refuse to speculate at all about motives. To this day, that is what I do. I don't speculate on why Governor Cuomo sentenced so many innocent frail elderly to death. I just know that is exactly what he did.

Second, you must not discount your own life experience. One of the things that has gone terribly wrong is the stampede to believe "expert" opinions. With two doctorate degrees after my name I certainly qualify as an expert and yet I am aware that most experts are misinforming you most of the time. Don't despair. If you want to know the truth about something, at this moment in human history, it is easier than ever to find the facts by carefully using the internet. But if you don't choose to become your own investigative reporter on a subject, do not discount your own life experience in favor of someone else's. Simply remain undecided. An example would be on masks.

If you are reading these words, then you have been living on this planet for somewhere between one to ten decades and during all of that time you have never believed holding a tissue or a cloth to your face stopped you from catching a cold or influenza. In the course of that time you have surely contracted a virus (probably a coronavirus) not knowing from where. In other words, thinking that a piece of cloth will keep you well contradicts all of your own life experience. Does this prove that masks are unnecessary? No. But the speed with which people have thrown away all their own life experience in favor of an expert's declaration is very problematic. Overwhelmingly, when the experts contradict your own life experience, the experts have been wrong.

Third, look for facts that existed prior to the controversy or dispute. What did the research say about masks or hydroxychloroquine prior to 2020? Ignore everything prior to the controversy and you will find the truth. Apply this rule going forward.

Fourth, do not listen to the opinions of the chattering class on cable news or social media until you have ascertained the facts for yourself. If you want to know about a policy or a policymaker, read the policy or listen to the policymaker before turning to commentary about them. Just like a parent who hears two versions of the same story from her two kids, the one you hear first sounds more plausible and neither version compares to seeing what happened yourself. For example, I don't believe anything posted on social media or the news. If something sounds interesting to me, I'll look for proof that it is true or false. The only exception is once I have personally ascertained that a particular source is trustworthy, I will return to that source. Reading social media is not harmless because in the process of absorbing random opinions, you erase the clean slate of your previously open mind.

Fifth, play a game of "20 questions" about the topic while pretending you don't have an opinion. This is not to land on a right or wrong judgment, but to test a news story or policy for authenticity. Factual stories tend to have any number of small, specific supporting details while inaccurate reports do not. On a topic you don't know, for which someone is trying to convince you, always ask for details. Truth has lots of supporting details.

Sixth, any conclusion that results in limiting your freedom must have a very high level of proof. Think of this like the difference in evidence required between a criminal case (potential jail time) and a civil matter, which does not involve jail time. In a criminal trial, the jury needs "proof beyond a reasonable doubt" which can be thought of as the jury being more than 90 percent certain, but in a civil proceeding the jury only needs a "preponderance of the evidence," or 51 percent certainty. All the lockdowns, closed businesses, closed schools, closed churches, masks, not being able to see your relatives—all of these things infringe on your freedom. They are not definitely always wrong, but when a politician suggests any solution that reduces freedom, you must require a very high level of proof.

Make a habit of thinking through issues using the six-point acronym MYPDQ-Freedom. Its common-sense-plus-critical-thinking approach will help you recognize disinformation before you are harmed by it.

MYPDQ-Freedom

Motives: ignore.

Your life experience: **don't ignore.**

Prior facts: known before the **controversy.**

Do not listen to the **chattering class.**

Questions: "20 questions" game shows the truth has many supporting details.

Freedom: laws limiting your freedom need a great deal of proof.

When people ask me today if I'll go back to being an emergency doctor the answer is unclear. Together with my family, the practice of medicine has defined my life. My immigrant father was a physician. He had an active practice, often seeing patients at our home. You might say I grew up in a doctor's office. Now I'm not sure if I'll ever return. I view my former colleagues as though through a long lens, far away. How can they not see what I see? I'm not sure I could ever be one of them again. It fills me with sadness to potentially leave behind the decades-long career that shaped my identity.

I pray that my story can inspire others to stand up for what they believe. We've seen the real-world costs of silence. Doctors couldn't freely practice medicine, and patients suffered. Many went without necessary care; tragically, so many died as a result. I watched the policy failures unfold before my own eyes, up close. There is no one aspect to these failures more important than any other. Yes, maligning and restricting hydroxychloroquine resulted in tens of thousands of unnecessary deaths. But other aspects were even more dehumanizing. As a society we were so quick to separate and marginalize people. Within a couple of weeks we isolated millions of frail elderly in nursing homes for months. No visitors, no therapy. This is infuriating and heartbreaking and this cannot be our national policy going forward.

Some emergency decrees have loosened, albeit only after considerable public outcry. If enough concerned citizens demand action from the people's representatives, more will follow. If enough doctors demand their independence and question shoddy science, more patients will be helped. America is an exceptional nation. Our history proves that we have a gift for learning from our mistakes and starting over. I did not consent to the conventional wisdom of elite opinion and neither should you.

The first White Coat Summit received close to twenty million views on social media within six to eight hours before being completely de-platformed. Had it stayed up it surely would have reached one hundred million views. The canceling of speech that Big Tech and Big Media dislike is known as "cancel culture." And it's rampant in our society.

The president of the United States of America re-tweeted the Summit and the president's own retweets were canceled by Twitter.

The CEO of Facebook decided that our words, speech, even our very persons were disinformation, and should be canceled by Facebook. Instagram, owned by Facebook, canceled the Summit. YouTube canceled the Summit. Squarespace, which hosted the domain, canceled the website.

The Declaration of Independence states that the government derives its powers from the consent of the governed. I do not consent to be governed by bureaucrats offering debunked conventional wisdom derived from a corrupt elite caste. Neither should you. You can find the original press conference and the hours of educational sessions on our new website, www.AmericasFrontlineDoctors.com.

Please sign up so that you are not censored from hearing the truth.

And finally, be joyful! We are blessed to live in an extraordinary country that has guaranteed our human freedom by law. While fighting to maintain this freedom, every one of us must enjoy our freedom. When you enjoy your freedom of speech, freedom of religion, freedom of assembly, you remind yourself and others **why we fight.**

Appendix

WHITE PAPER ON HYDROXYCHLOROQUINE

Synopsis:

This white paper is to draw the reader's attention to the indisputable safety of hydroxychloroquine (HCQ), an analog of the same quinine found in tree barks that George Washington used to protect his troops. The modern version has been FDA approved for 65 years, has shown remarkable efficacy against SARS-CoV-2 and its use is being wrongly restricted despite the immediate danger to the American people and the rest of the world.

We speak in support of immediately reversing the massive, irresponsible disinformation campaign that is literally preventing doctors from dispensing HCQ, advocating as well that it be made available over the counter in the United States. This is logistically easy to do in a manner that ensures the supply and appropriate dispensation.

Introduction:

The purpose of this white paper is to dispassionately present the evidence regarding the safety and efficacy of hydroxychloroquine and determine its proper role in the current pandemic.

General Consensus that Hydroxychloroquine is Safe

Hydroxychloroquine (HCQ) has been FDA approved for over 65 years and has been used billions of times throughout the entire world without restriction. For many decades it has been given to: pregnant women, breastfeeding women, children, elderly patients, immune compromised patients and healthy persons.

In the USA it is used most often in three situations: systemic lupus erythematosus (SLE), rheumatoid arthritis (RA), and as malaria prophylaxis for travelers. These three situations happen to represent three different types of populations.

> Patients with SLE are immune compromised.
> Patients with RA are elderly.
> Travelers are younger and typically healthy.

Although all doctors can and do prescribe HCQ, because it is most commonly used for SLE and RA, **rheumatology** specialists are the physicians in America who prescribe it the most. Although it is in the safest category of medication and it is virtually always safely used, the two most common possible complications fall under the specialty of **cardiology** and **ophthalmology**.

So let us see what these three types of specialties say.

What do the Rheumatologists Say?

The physicians who prescribe HCQ the most are **rheu-matologists**. Patients who need HCQ typically are on the medication for years or decades. Therefore rheumatologists have extensive experience with this medication. They make decisions daily regarding this medication. They decide who can get the medication, is safe or unsafe, how much to give, how often to dose, when to increase/decrease the dose, what testing if any should be done prior to starting the medication, can the medicine be taken with other medicines, when to stop the medication, what the side effects are. To help them with such decisions, rheumatologists can check with their professional society: American College of Rheumatology (ACR.)

The ACR website:

> Hydroxychloroquine typically is very well tolerated. Serious side effects are rare. The most common side effects are nausea and diarrhea, which often improve with time. Less common side effects include rash, changes in skin pigment (such as darkening or dark spots), hair changes, and muscle weakness. Rarely, hydroxychloroquine can lead to anemia in some individuals. This can happen in individuals with a condition known as G6PD deficiency or porphyria.

> In rare cases, hydroxychloroquine can cause visual changes or loss of vision. Such vision problems are more likely to occur in individuals taking high doses for many years, in individuals

60 years or older, those with significant kidney or liver disease, and those with underlying retinal disease. At the recommended dose, development of visual problems due to the medication is rare. It is recommended that you have an eye exam within the first year of use, then repeat every 1 to 5 years based on current guidelines.

Additional rare reports of changes in the heart rhythm have been reported with the use of hydroxychloroquine, particularly in combination with other medications. While monitoring for this risk is not typical in the office setting, it has been indicated in hospitalized and critically ill patients to evaluate for interactions with other medications.[1]

In other words the professional society of the physicians who prescribe this drug the most, for years have said the following:
1. serious side effects are rare
2. visual changes can happen in people taking high doses for years
3. heart rhythm changes are so uncommon that there is no monitoring pre-use

In an interview with Dr. Mehmet Oz, prominent Los Angeles rheumatologist, Professor of Medicine, Associate Director of the Rheumatology Dept. Cedars Sinai Medical Center Dr. Daniel Wallace said the following:[2]

1   https://www.rheumatology.org/Portals/0/Files/Hydroxychloro-quine-Plaquenil-Fact-Sheet.pdf?ver=2020-04-30-154904-073

2   https://www.youtube.com/watch?v=htyCEeq_YVI

Dr. Oz: Is HCQ safe?
A: In 42 years of clinical practice I've treated several thousand lupus patients and I would like to emphasize that all rheumatologists have a great deal of experience with this drug. Regarding safety, since it came out 70 years ago, several million patients have taken the drug. There have not been any reported deaths from using this agent as monotherapy or taken only by itself.

Dr. Oz: Q: arrhythmia, heart issues?
A: It is a problem with CQ, which is its first cousin. And it *was* a problem with HCQ in the 1950's and 1960's when doctors were using 2-3x its usual dose. In the current recommended dose it really does not occur. 400 mg/day.

What do the Cardiologists Say?

Next let us consider the alleged complication that has dominated the news, which is a potential heart problem. Those specialists are cardiologists. Heart rhythm problems are so rare with HCQ that it is common practice not to do an EKG prior to starting the medication. It's the opposite of the truth to claim that there is a heart risk when the specialty professional organization denies that, and when it is not what has been done for decades prior to this pandemic. In addition, the American Heart Association has demonstrated it is safe during Covid-19, which will be discussed below.[3]

---

3   https://www.ahajournals.org/doi/10.1161/CIRCEP.120.008662

Prominent Los Angeles cardiologist Dr. Daniel Wohlgelernter states:

> Over the last 30 years I have had several hundred patient visits specifically to discuss the toxicity of hydroxychloroquine. During that time, not a single patient has been taken off of this drug for cardiac toxicity.[4]

The largest meta analysis published in 2018, revealed only 50 cardiac deaths attributed to hydroxychloroquine in 60 plus years.[5]

The largest database analysis that examined this issue stated the following:

> The results on the risk of severe adverse events associated with short-term (1 month) HCQ treatment as proposed for COVID-19 therapy are reassuring, with no excess risk of any of the considered safety outcomes compared to an equivalent therapy.[6]

What do the Ophthalmologists Say?

In an interview with Laura Ingraham, Dr. Richard Urso, ophthalmologist said this:

> I have had several thousand patient visits to specifically discuss the toxicity of this drug over

---

4   http://www.santamonicacardiology.com/wohlgelernter.php

5   https://pubmed.ncbi.nlm.nih.gov/29858838/?from_term=Hydroxychloroquine+and+cardiac&from_pos=1

6   https://www.medrxiv.org/content/10.1101/2020.04.08.20054551v2

my last 30 years. It's a super safe drug. It's safer than Tylenol, aspirin, Motrin.[7]

There is no visual risk for short courses of HCQ. No one ever even suggests such a thing. The people who use HCQ for a short period of time are travelers. Even the CDC website does not suggest an eye exam. Rheumatologists and ophthalmologists who are familiar with the rare visual problems all say the same thing. There is a rare risk of retinopathy that is possible when a patient has been on the medication for many years. The risk of retinal toxicity at five years of continuous use is zero. The risk of retinal toxicity at ten years of continuous use is 1%. It gets higher after ten years of continuous use."[8]

Toxicity can be seen in the macula and electrical conduction of the heart, after years of use. Typically patients who have ingested 1/2 to 1 kilo in their lifetime become more susceptible to these issues. Over a short-term course it is never seen.[9]

To put the amount that is needed to even possibly be at risk for retinopathy in perspective, that is many years of using daily.

Safety Studies

It is self-evident that HCQ is safe from the fact that it has been FDA approved for 65 years and has been used many billions of times all over the world and it is over the counter

---

7   Dr. Richard Urso, ophthalmologist on Laura Ingraham July 10, 2020.

8   Dr. Daniel Wallace, rheumatologist on Dr. Oz April 8, 2020 https://www.youtube.com/watch?v=htyCEeq_YVI

9   Dr. Richard Urso, ophthalmologist on Laura Ingraham July 10, 2020

in most of the world, certainly pre-2020. It is the #1 most used medication in India, the second most populous nation on the planet with 1.3 billion people. If an American travels to a location where malaria is endemic, per the CDC, they would start HCQ before they left for their trip. There has never been an allegation that HCQ is not safe until 2020.

The only allegations of HCQ not being safe relate to a potential heart problem. The media has stated this so often that many people, including physicians, think there is a potential heart problem. However the evidence is overwhelming that HCQ is very low risk.

I. In the largest study to date on the subject, HCQ has been shown to not increase heart (cardiac) risk.[10] This study was across a multinational, distributed database network. It studied all the data for 20 years, from January 9, 2000 – 2020 on patients who were prescribed HCQ. The study had two goals: to understand the safety of HCQ by itself and its safety when paired with the antibiotic azithromycin. This paper was authored by scientists from 33 countries and companies across the world.

---

10 https://www.medrxiv.org/content/10.1101/2020.04.08.20054551v2. The authors include scientists from: University of Oxford, Fundacio Institut Universitari per a la recerca a l'Atencio Primaria de Salut Jordi Gol I Gurina, University of Sao Paulo, Massachusetts General Hospital, King Saud University, Harvard School of Public Health, Department of Veterans Affairs, University of Utah School of Medicine, University of Zagreb School of Medicine, Columbia University Medical Center, Islamic University of Gaza, New York Presbyterian Hospital, National Institute for Health and Care UK, University of New Mexico Health Sciences Center, Erasmus Medical Center, Vanderbilt University, University of Arizona College of Medicine, University of Dundee Scotland, Institute of Medicine Sweden, Ajou University South Korea, National University of Singapore, UCLA, Shanghai University of Traditional Chinese Medicine, Peking Union Medical College, University of Melbourne, Janssen Research, Real World Solution, Actelion Pharmaceuticals, Real-World Evidence Spain, AstraZeneca, RTI Health Solutions, Bayer Pharmaceuticals

The paper is titled "Safety of hydroxychloroquine, alone and in combination with azithromycin, in light of rapid widespread use for COVID-19: a multinational, network cohort and self-controlled case series study." In plain English, the authors found that over a twenty-year period, looking at almost one million patients, those taking HCQ did not have an increased risk of heart problems. It says:

> This is the largest ever analysis of the safety of such treatments worldwide, examining over 900,000 HCQ and more than 300,000 HCQ + azithromycin users respectively. The results on the risk of serious adverse events associated with short-term (1 month) HCQ treatment as proposed for COVID-19 therapy are reassuring, with no excess risk of any of the considered safety outcomes compared to an equivalent therapy.

II. The FDA database shows a total of 640 deaths attributable to HCQ over fifty years. To put this in context "Each year the FDA receives over one million adverse event reports associated with the use of drug products" "This concerns the entirety of HCQ use over more than 50 years of data, likely millions of uses and of longer-term use than the five days recommended for Covid-19 treatment."[11] The 640 deaths represented 0.034% of all the deaths (1,910,212) attributable to medications.

---

11 US Food & Drug Administration. FDA Adverse Events Reporting System (FAERS) Public Dashboard. https://fis.fda.gov/sense/app/d10be6bb-494e-4cd2-82e4-0135608ddc13/sheet/7a47a261-d58b-4203-a8aa-6d3021737452/state/analysis

III. <u>The CDC has an information sheet about HCQ</u>. That sheet includes the following questions/answers.[12]

Q: Who can take hydroxychloroquine?
A: Hydroxychloroquine can be prescribed to adults and children of all ages. It can also be safely taken by pregnant women and nursing mothers.

Q: Who should not take hydroxychloroquine?
A: People with psoriasis should not take hydroxychloroquine.

Q: How should I take hydroxychloroquine?
A: Both adults and children should take one dose of hydroxychloroquine per week <u>starting at least one week before</u> traveling... They should take one dose per week while there, and for <u>four consecutive weeks after</u> leaving. **The weekly dosage for adults in 400 mg.**

Q: What are the potential side effects of hydroxychloroquine?
A: Hydroxychloroquine is a relatively well tolerated medicine. The most common adverse reactions reported are stomach pain, nausea, vomiting, and headache. These side effects can often be lessened by taking hydroxychloroquine with food. Hydroxychloroquine may also cause itching in some people.

---

12 https://www.cdc.gov/parasites/malaria/index.html

Q: How long is it safe to use hydroxychloroquine?

A: CDC has no limits on the use of hydroxychloroquine for the prevention of malaria. When hydroxychloroquine is used at higher doses for many years, a rare eye condition called retinopathy has occurred. People who take hydroxychloroquine for more than five years should get regular eye exams.

IV. <u>It is well established that there is no scientific basis for the claim that HCQ is risky on its own</u>. The only credible theory as to why there has even been a concern, is that since the beginning, possible treatment options of COVID-19 have always included HCQ in *combination* with the antibiotic azithromycin. Because each medication independently can cause the same rare heart rhythm disturbance, there has been an academic concern whether the two drugs could be risky when taken together. The particular heart rhythm problem is called "QT prolongation" and it is a known side effect of hundreds of drugs. If the "QT prolongation" is severe it can lead to a fatal rhythm problem called Torsades de Pointes. Even though it is rare, this has been alleged to be of serious and frequent enough concern that people should not use HCQ for Covid-19. The American Heart Association has now answered this specific question. (April 29, 2020)

> In the largest reported cohort of coronavirus disease 2019 to date treated with chloroquine/ hydroxychloroquine +/- azithromycin, **no** instances of Torsades de Pointes or arrhythmogenic death were reported.[13]

---

13 https://www.ahajournals.org/doi/10.1161/CIRCEP.120.008662

In plain English: Taking HCQ even in combination with the antibiotic azithromycin does not cause an increased risk of ~~fatal heart rhythm problems.~~

The most comprehensive study on the subject was authored by Dr. Harvey Risch, MD, PhD, Professor of Epidemiology at Yale School of Public Health, and published in affiliation with the Johns Hopkins Bloomberg School of Public Health.[14] Dr. Risch who has 39,779 citations on Google Scholar, reviewed five outpatient studies, and shows with specificity how the results have been misinterpreted, misstated and misreported. He notes the following.

> 1. When examining the data on safety, Dr. Risch notes that early evidence of safety was being ignored. "Lack of any cardiac arrhythmia events in the 405 Zelenko patients or the 1061 Marseilles patients or the 412 Brazil patients."

> 2. When examining the data on safety, Dr. Risch demonstrates that the negative conclusions drawn by various professional organizations are not based upon science. "It is unclear why the FDA, NIH, and cardiology societies made their [negative] recommendations about HCQ+AZM use now, when the Oxford study analyzed 323,122 users of HCQ+AZ … that the combination of HCQ+AZ has been in widespread standard-of-care use in the US and elsewhere for decades … this use predominantly in

---

14 https://www.aspph.org/yale-dr-harvey-risch-wins-50000-ruth-leff-siegel-award/

older adults with multiple comorbidities, with no such strident warnings about the use given during that time."[15]

Efficacy

There are only two things that must be considered regarding a medication: is it safe and does it work? HCQ is amongst the safest of all prescription drugs in USA and that is why across much of the world it is sold over the counter. And at a time when the world has become seized with panic over a virus without a specific cure, the question of effectiveness is almost moot. If a drug is safe and might work, and if there are no other options, we must try it.

The safety record of HCQ is indisputable. But now seven months into the pandemic there is overwhelming evidence accumulating that HCQ is also *effective* for Covid-19. There are dozens of studies demonstrating its effectiveness from all around the world. From China to France to Saudi Arabia to Iran to Italy to India to New York City to Michigan to Brazil. This is not surprising. As far back as, chloroquine (CQ) the first cousin of HCQ and previously known to be effective against SARS-CoV-1, was stated by China to be a treatment for Covid-19.

> • February 19, 2020 China: "The drug [chloroquine] is recommended to be included in the next version of the Guidelines for the Prevention, Diagnosis, and Treatment of Pneumonia Caused by COVID-19 issued by the National Health Commission of the Peo-

---

15 https://www.medrxiv.org/content/10.1101/2020.04.08.20054551v2

ple's Republic of China for the treatment of COVID-10 infection in larger populations in the future."[16]

• March 4, 2020: France: "The first results obtained from more than 100 patients show the superiority of chloroquine compared with treatment of the control group in terms of reduction of exacerbation of pneumonia, duration of symptoms and delay of viral clearance all in the absence of severe side effects."[17]

• March 20, 2020: New York: 1450 patients. 1045 mild and not requiring meds (all recovered), 405 treated with HCQ + AZM + Zinc of which six were hospitalized and two died.[18]

• March 22, 2020: India: The country of India recommends HCQ prophylaxis broadly.[19]

• March 22, 2020: China: "Among patients with Covid-19, HCQ could significantly shorten time to complete recovery and promote the absorption of pneumonia."[20]

• April 11, 2020: France: All patients [treated with HCQ + AZM] improved clinically ex-

16 https://www.jstage.jst.go.jp/article/bst/14/1/14_2020.01047/_article

17 https://www.ncbi.nlm.nih.gov/pmc/articles/PMC7135139/

18 https://academic.oup.com/aje/article/doi/10.1093/aje/kwaa093/5847586

19 https://www.mohfw.gov.in/pdf/AdvisoryontheuseofHydroxychloroquinasprophylaxisforSARSCoV2infection.pdf

20 https://www.medrxiv.org/content/10.1101/2020.03.22.20040758v3

cept [two]... A rapid fall of nasopharyngeal viral load was noted. ... Patients were able to be rapidly discharged from IDU [Infectious Disease Unit]..." [21]

• April 13, 2020: NY: 54 long-term care/ nursing home patients received HCQ+ Doxycycline and only 5.6% died. (this population can have >50% mortality) [22] [23]

• April 17, 2020: Brazil: Of 636 symptomatic high-risk outpatients, only 1.9% of those treated needed hospitalization vs., 5.4% of the untreated. [24]

• April 21, 2020: 16 countries: "The difference in dynamics of daily deaths is so striking that we believe that the urgency context commands presenting the analysis ..."[25] [26]

• April 24, 2020: Iran: Hydroxychloroquine ...can be potential treatment options.[27]

• April 30, 2020: Saudi Arabia: "Chloroquine

21 https://www.sciencedirect.com/science/article/pii/S1477893920301319

22 ABC News. https://abc7ny.com/coronavirus-treatment-long-island-news-nassau-county/6093072/

23 https://pubmed.ncbi.nlm.nih.gov/32418114/

24 https://pgibertie.files.wordpress.com/2020/04/2020.04.15-journal-manuscript-final.pdf

25 https://papers.ssrn.com/sol3/papers.cfm?abstract_id=3575899

26 https://www.medrxiv.org/content/10.1101/2020.04.18.20063875v2

27 https://www.researchgate.net/publication/341197843_COVID-19_in_Iran_a_comprehensive_investigation_from_exposure_to_treatment_outcomes

and hydroxychloroquine have antiviral characteristics in vitro. The findings support the hypotheses that these drugs have efficacy in the treatment of COvid-19."[28]

• May 15, 2020: China: We found that fatalities are 18.8% in the HCQ group, significantly lower than 47.4% in the non-HCQ group. These data demonstrate that addition of HCQ on top of the basic treatments is highly effective in reducing the fatality of critically ill patients of Covid-19 through attenuation of inflammatory cytokine storm. Therefore, HCQ should be prescribed as a part of treatment for critically ill Covid-19 patients, with possible outcome of saving lives. [29]

• May 16, 2020: France: 1061 Covid-positive patients treated with HCQ+AZM "no cardiac toxicity was observed" and "good clinical outcome and virological cure were seen in 92%.[30]

• June 6, 2020: France: "In conclusion, a meta-analysis of publicly available clinical reports demonstrates that chloroquine ... reduces mortality by a factor 3 in patients infected with Covid-19."[31]

---

28 https://www.europeanreview.org/wp/wp-content/uploads/4539-4547.pdf

29 https://pubmed.ncbi.nlm.nih.gov/32418114/

30 https://www.mediterranee-infection.com/wp-content/uploads/2020/04/MS.pdf

31 https://www.sciencedirect.com/science/article/pii/S2052297520300615?via%3Dihub

• June 20, 2020: India: "Consumption of four or more maintenance doses of HCQ was associated with a significant decline in the odds of getting infected… This study provides actionable information for policy-makers to protect healthcare workers at the forefront of Covid-19 response."[32] [33]

• June 29, 2020: Portugal: The odds ration of [Covid-19] infection in patient with chronic treatment with HCQ is half.[34]

• June 29, 2020: Detroit: "In this multi-hospital assessment, when controlling for Covid-19 risk factors, treatment with HCQ alone and in combination with AZM was associated with reduction in Covid-19 mortality."[35]

• June 30, 2020: NYC: 6493 patients who had laboratory confirmed Covid-19 with clinical outcomes between March 13-April 17, 2020 who were seen in 8 hospitals and 400 clinics in the NYC metropolitan area. "Hydroxychloroquine use was associated with decreased mortality."[36]

32 http://www.ijmr.org.in/article.asp?issn=0971-5916;year=2020;volume=151;issue=5;spage=459;epage=467;aulast=Chatterjee

33 https://www.ncbi.nlm.nih.gov/research/coronavirus/publication/32611916

34 https://www.medrxiv.org/content/10.1101/2020.06.26.20056507v1

35 https://www.ijidonline.com/action/showPdf?pii=S1201-9712%2820%2930534-8

36 https://link.springer.com/article/10.1007/s11606-020-05983-z

- <u>July 3, 2020</u>: NY: Covid-positive patients treated with HCQ + AZM + Zinc vs. untreated.[37]

  - hospitalized: treated 2.8% vs. untreated 15.4%
  - death: treated 0.7% vs. untreated 3.5%
  - No cardiac side effects
  - 5x less all-cause deaths

- <u>August 20, 2020:</u> NJ: 1274 outpatients with documented SARS-CoV-2 found HCQ exposure cut hospitalization from 31% to 21% and cut mortality in half and no HCQ patient had arrhythmia-event.[38]

As discussed in the Safety section, the most comprehensive study on the subject was authored by Dr. Harvey Risch, MD, PhD, Professor of Epidemiology at Yale School of Public Health, and published in affiliation with the Johns Hopkins Bloomberg School of Public Health.[39] He notes the following.

1. When examining data on efficacy, Dr. Risch notes that the French studies were routinely disparaged as not being randomized, controlled and double-blinded. (Although that is the gold standard in research, it is of course

---

37 https://www.preprints.org/manuscript/202007.0025/v1

38 https://www.medrxiv.org/content/10.1101/2020.08.20.20178772v1.full.pdf

39 https://www.aspph.org/yale-dr-harvey-risch-wins-50000-ruth-leff-siegel-award/

impossible in the beginning stages of investigating a new disease.) However Dr. Risch notes that the results were so stunning as to far outweigh that issue. "The first study of HCQ + AZM showed a 50x benefit vs. standard of care. This is such an enormous difference that it cannot be ignored despite lack of randomization."[40]

2. When examining data on efficacy, Dr. Risch notes that **evidence against HCQ when it is used alone is irrelevant, as it has been known since Feb-March that HCQ must be used in combination therapy.**[41]

Four Levels of Obfuscation Used to Disparage This Remedy

Corruption of the Scientific Journals

It is well known that **The Lancet** and **The New England Journal of Medicine** (NEJM) had to retract their studies. It was well documented in a series published in The Guardian starting with the headline: "The Lancet has made one of the biggest retractions in modern history. How could this happen?"[42] The sheer number and magnitude of the things

---

40 Gautret P, Lagier J-C, Parola P, et al. Hydroxychlorquine and azithromycin as a treatment of Covid-19: results of an open-label non-randomized clinical trial. Int J Antimicrob Agent 2020 Mar 17. https://pubmed.ncbi.nlm.nih.gov/32205204/

41 https://stopcovid19.today/wp-content/uploads/2020/04/COVID_19_RAPPORT_ETUDE_RETROSPECTIVE_CLINIQUE_ET_THERAPEU-TIQUE_200430.pdf

42 https://www.theguardian.com/commentisfree/2020/jun/05/lancet-had-to-do-one-of-the-biggest-retractions-in-modern-history-how-could-this-happen

that went wrong or missing are too enormous to attribute to mere incompetence.

The data upon which these studies were based were so ridiculously erroneous that it only took two weeks for an eagle-eyed physician to publicly demand an explanation.[43] What's incredible is that the editors of these esteemed journals still have a job – that is how utterly incredible the supposed data underlying the studies was. The company that "gathered" the alleged data (Surgisphere) is now wiped clean from the Internet.

The Lancet and The NEJM have at least been exposed, but the third premier journal, as yet unexposed, is the **Journal of the American Medical Association** (JAMA.) While the first two journals published fraudulent studies, the JAMA study seems criminal in its utter disregard for human life.

The worldwide fallout from these three journals was fast and furious:

> USA Today: "Coronavirus Patients who took HCQ had higher risk of death, study shows."[44]

> The World Health Organization ordered nations to stop using HCQ and CQ,[45] WHO Chief Tedros suspended trials being held in hundreds of hospitals across the world,[46]

---

43 https://www.youtube.com/watch?v=4HYK5pL2Z_s

44 https://www.usatoday.com/story/news/health/2020/05/22/covid-19-study-links-hydroxychloroquine-higher-risk-death/5244664002/

45 https://www.reuters.com/article/us-health-coronavirus-indonesia-chloroqu/exclusive-indonesia-major-advocate-of-hydroxychloroquine-told-by-who-to-stop-using-it-idUSKBN23227L

46 https://medicalxpress.com/news/2020-05-trial-hydroxychloro-

The EU governments France, Italy, and Belgium banned HCQ for Covid-19 trials,[47]

Worldwide ridicule was heaped upon the President of the United States.[48][49]
One can speculate how it is possible that the #1, #2, and #3 most famous medical journals in the world have jointly, erroneously, and virtually simultaneously, condemned HCQ/CQ. Here is one theory.

Dr. Dousty-Blazy, the former French Health Minister, Under Secretary General of UN, and candidate for Director of WHO has publicly stated that The Lancet and the NEJM Editors admit to being pressured by pharmaceutical companies to publish certain results.

> The Lancet's boss ... said ... the pharmaceutical companies are so financially powerful today and are able to use such methodologies as to have us accept papers which ... in reality manage to conclude what they want ... I have been doing research for 20 years of my life. I never thought the boss of The Lancet could say that. And the boss of the NEJM too. He even said it was 'criminal.'[50]

---

quine-covid-treatment.html

47 https://www.reuters.com/article/health-coronavirus-hydroxychloro-quine-fr/eu-governments-ban-malaria-drug-for-covid-19-trial-paused-as-safety-fears-grow-idUSKBN2340A6

48 https://www.nytimes.com/2020/05/18/us/politics/trump-hydroxychloro-quine-covid-coronavirus.html

49 https://www.nytimes.com/2020/05/22/health/malaria-drug-trump-coro-navirus.html

50 https://www.youtube.com/watch?v=ZYgiCALEdpE

In the case of the JAMA study, the scientists gave up to 2.5x lethal dosage of the medication.[51] Unsurprisingly so many patients died they halted the study early. They also cherry-picked patients and had no proof that there was the standard ethics oversight of the study. JAMA knew of these problems and published the study anyway. Various scientists have demanded its retraction, and even now, with civil and *criminal* investigations into these deaths, the study is still is not retracted. And the headlines around this study blame the drug, not the fact that old, sick, hospitalized, compromised patients were given toxic dosages of a drug.

This is a mockery. These journals did not publish science, but instead published fiction or evidence of a crime.

Corruption of the Media

In addition to the corruption of the Journals we must note the widespread disinformation campaign as regards this safe and effective medication. While we don't blame individual journalists or publishers, in the aggregate, it is breathtaking that the overwhelming news regarding HCQ is positive and yet it is almost impossible to find any good news in the American media.

For example at approximately the same time The Lancet and the NEJM and JAMA published their retracted and possibly criminal studies, one of the oldest and most prestigious Journals in the world, the Indian Journal of Medical Research published very good news regarding HCQ.[52] Few

---

51 https://jamanetwork.com/journals/jamacardiology/fullarticle/2765631

52 http://www.ijmr.org.in/article.asp?issn=0971-5916;year=2020;volume=151;issue=5;spage=459;epage=467;aulast=Chatterjee

have heard of this study because the mainstream press has ignored it.

Another example is the inexplicable delay in the publication of the Detroit study. This study was completed May 2, 2020."[53] The Detroit study was not published until just before the July 4th Holiday and there was also no pre-publication press conference hinting at the good news. In normal times, a lag of seven weeks would be acceptable, but the Detroit results were showed a half mortality rate and everything regarding Covid-19 era is published at warp speed. Why the delay?

Censorship of the Public "Town Square"

The clearest example of physician free speech censorship is what happened to James Todaro, MD.[54] Dr. Todaro, who up until these events was a mere private citizen, tweeted his thoughts about HCQ including a link to a public Google doc six days *before* the President endorsed HCQ. Dr. Todaro's apolitical scientific commentary was his opinion of a scientific study that appeared to be fabricated, despite being published in a world-class journal. It turns out Dr. Todaro was so spot-on *correct,* that the study, which unfortunately had enormous worldwide influence, was *retracted* which is exceedingly rare. But before the public could read Dr. Todaro's prescient words, the President happened to endorse HCQ, and Google scrubbed the document within hours.

---

53 https://www.ijidonline.com/action/showPdf?pii
=S1201-9712%2820%2930534-8

54 https://docs.google.com/document/d/1HY50zIjuSIVKltTk5UegfgqdiH-
N9ehLxLqLES9nwDZ8/edit?ts=5f106ac5

And by scrubbed we mean that Google didn't want you to think it was *missing*, they wanted you to not know such a thing ever even *existed*. This is how is happens.

First, Dr. Todaro has already learned that he will be censored, so he decides to bypass the censor by not even attempting to get a mainstream news source to publish his story about HCQ. He has accepted that even though his story is exactly the kind of counter-culture story that used to be sought after by journalists, those days are gone.

So Dr. Todaro self-publishes a document that he wrote and puts it out for public view, on a site that calls itself content-neutral: Google. Google claims it is a platform and not a publisher, which is a huge distinction. Platforms are just the vehicle to get the words from point a to point b. Publishers are responsible for content. If Google is a platform, which it represents itself to be, including before Congress, then it should not censor non-salacious content written by a scientist about science.

Censorship is evident for those who wish to see it.

Excessive & Punitive Regulations at the State Level & "Off-Label" Prescribing

There is obviously a tremendous disinformation campaign going on in the United States of America claiming that HCQ is neither safe nor effective. This is quite remarkable for a medication that has been FDA approved for 65 years and having already been dispensed billions of times all across the world with only 57 serious adverse events (heart) noted by the FDA in their own database over the past fifty years. In many countries it is available over the counter, like aspirin and Tylenol.

Nonetheless, with the negative pressure being applied, state Governors have ordered, through their state licensing boards that physicians stop using it, and pharmacists stop dispensing it. Their wording is often more cautious, but doctors are told that they could be charged with "unprofessional conduct" (a threat to their license) or be "sanctioned" if they prescribe. First we need to understand how prescriptions have been done for decades.

Once approved by the FDA, any physician can prescribe any prescription medication in the USA, for any reason.[55] This is significant in that a drug is not approved for a specific diagnosis; a drug either makes it through the years-long approval process or it does not. That means a medication can be used "on-label" (the reason it was approved) or "off-label" (other reasons that have never received FDA approval.) It costs a lot of money for the pharmaceutical company to gain another "on-label" use, so once a drug is approved for any use, it is typically used for many reasons. Those additional reasons are called "off-label."

As a practical matter "off-label" use accounts for about 20% of prescriptions. It is a daily occurrence. For example, it is off-label to give morphine as a pain medication for children. Indomethacin (an anti-inflammatory) was discovered in the 1970's to work for a specific heart condition in newborns and is the standard of care for that condition (PDA) even though it has *never* been approved for this diagnosis. The very popular anti-nausea drug "Zofran" is given routinely (doctors call it the "bacon" of drugs) for virtually any type of nausea but it only has two very specific on-label indications: post-operative and chemotherapy induced nausea.

---

55 https://www.ncbi.nlm.nih.gov/pmc/articles/PMC3538391/

Another very common example is aspirin, which is *not* indicated for heart (coronary artery disease) prophylaxis in diabetics and yet it is the formal recommendation and standard practice by cardiologists.[56] It has been estimated that 73% of off-label use had low or no scientific support.[57] Pediatric antidepressant drugs are typically used off-label and are prone to error.[58]

There is a complete disconnect between physicians and everyone else on the subject of off-label use.[59] While almost all members of the public have benefited from "off-label" use of drug, many may not be focused on the distinction between "off-label" and "on-label" usages. This is logical as patients rely on and know physicians are personally and professionally obligated (and subject to much oversight and malpractice litigation), to do what is in the patient's best interest.

Exploiting the public's understandable lack of focus on the non-distinction between off-label and on-label has contributed to the public's confusion regarding HCQ for Covid-19. From the physician's perspective if a drug is FDA approved and safe it is within the physician's armamentarium. And from the physician's perspective, is highly suspect that that rule should change in the middle of a pandemic and without any legislative discussion or regulation whatsoever, let

---

56 Regulating off-label drug use--rethinking the role of the FDA. *Stafford RS N Engl J Med. 2008 Apr 3; 358(14):1427-9.*

57 Off-label prescribing among office-based physicians. *Radley DC, Finkelstein SN, Stafford RS Arch Intern Med. 2006 May 8; 166(9):1021-*

58 Pediatric antidepressant medication errors in a national error reporting database. *Rinke ML, Bundy DG, Shore AD, Colantuoni E, Morlock LL, Miller MR J Dev Behav Pediatr. 2010 Feb-Mar; 31(2):129-36.*

59 https://www.wsj.com/articles/SB116422408807730936

alone sound science to support the same. It has **never** happened that a state has threatened a doctor for prescribing a universally accepted safe generic cheap drug off-label.

Although the states are the entities that empower physicians to prescribe, examples of abusive state actions will be in the next (federal) section because the states commonly blame the FDA (federal) for their newly aggressive regulations. But please note that many doctors have personally attested to the four harms caused by these Governors/State Medical Boards.[60]

1. doctors have been sanctioned, disciplined, interrogated
2. pharmacists have been empowered to override physicians
3. patients get sicker and die
4. physicians self-censoring due to fear of retribution

Misstatements at the Federal (FDA) Level

Hydroxychloroquine is safe as a matter of fact, as demonstrated above. It is also considered "legally" safe as a matter of law as it is FDA approved for 65 years and doctors have been freely prescribing it in all that time until Covid-19. Contradicting its own policy, we believe for the first time in its history, the FDA has made statements that have caused states to restrict its use. While the right to prescribe is granted by each state, the states are informed by the FDA, and in reliance on the FDA, here are examples of over-reaching by many states.

---

60 https://aapsonline.org/judicial/aaps-v-fda-hcq-6-2-2020.pdf

Arkansas:[61]
Updated June 16, 2020

The Food and Drug Administration (FDA) has announced the removal of Emergency Use Authorizations (EUA) for chloroquine (CQ) and hydroxychloroquine (HCQ) to treat COVID-19. The announcement follows the FDA's determination that CQ and HCQ are unlikely effective treatments for COVID-19. In addition, the FDA further indicated the potential benefit does not outweigh the potential serious cardiovascular events and other adverse effects that can be caused by CQ and HCQ.2

Based on this information, the Arkansas Department of Health has updated its guidance related to hydroxychloroquine and chloroquine. The utilization of CQ and HCQ for treatment of COVID-19 should be avoided in both outpatient and hospitalized settings. HCQ that has been distributed through the Strategic National Stockpile is no longer authorized under the EUA to treat hospitalized patients for COVID-19, unless they had already started treatments.

Chloroquine and hydroxychloroquine should be administered, prescribed and dispensed for FDA approved medical conditions under supervision of a patient's healthcare provider.

---

61 https://www.healthy.arkansas.gov/programs-services/topics/covid-19-guidance-about-chloroquine

California:[62]

Statement Regarding Improper Prescribing of Medications Related to Treatment for Novel Coronavirus (COVID-19)

Several states have recently issued emergency restrictions on how the drugs can be dispensed. Many require that medications be prescribed and dispensed only to patients with a legitimate and current medical condition. Further, the FDA recently issued an Emergency Use Authorization to allow for the use of hydroxychloroquine sulfate and chloroquine phosphate products donated by the Strategic National Stockpile for certain hospitalized patients with COVID-19.

DCA, the Medical Board of California, and the California State Board of Pharmacy remind health care professionals that inappropriately prescribing or dispensing medications constitutes unprofessional conduct in California. Prescribers and pharmacists are obligated to follow the law, standard of care, and professional codes of ethics in serving their patients and public health.

Colorado:[63]

Here are recommendations, first distributed by The American Society of Health-System Pharmacists (ASHP) to its membership, which may serve as a

---

62 Author has original copy

63 https://content.govdelivery.com/accounts/CODORA/bulletins/2833740

general guide for healthcare professionals regarding the receipt and dispensing of prescriptions for hydroxychloroquine, which can be applied to other COVID-19 investigative medications.

1. Continue to fill prescriptions for existing patients who are being prescribed these medications for FDA-approved indications on chronic therapy.

2. For new prescriptions, prescribers should be cognizant that hydroxychloroquine use in COVID-19 patients is not the standard of care. Pharmacists should verify and document diagnosis with the prescriber or prescriber's agent and limit to a 30-day supply of medication with the drug frequently on back order at this time for prescriptions with an FDA-approved indication.

3. Due to limited supply, reserve hydroxychloroquine for patients with known autoimmune disorders and those ill enough to be hospitalized for COVID-19.

Please note that the Colorado State Board of Pharmacy, the Colorado Medical Board and the Colorado Nursing Board have the authority to discipline their corresponding licensees who fail to meet their corresponding generally accepted standards of practice.

Connecticut:[64]

DPH strongly advises against off-label use of hydroxychloroquine and azithromycin in the outpatient setting for COVID-19 prophylaxis or treatment.

New Hampshire:[65]

Chloroquine, hydroxychloroquine, and albuterol inhalers shall be subject to the following controls, restrictions, and rationing: a) Outpatient prescriptions for patients not already established on chloroquine and hydroxychloroquine shall be limited to a 30-day supply. b) No prescriptions of chloroquine or hydroxychloroquine shall be issued or dispensed as prophylaxis treatment for COVID-19. c) Prescribing providers, when issuing a prescription in any form for chloroquine or hydroxychloroquine, must document an indication for all patients, including patients already established on these medications. d) For albuterol inhalers, prescribing providers shall limit prescriptions to one inhaler with up to three refills for all new prescriptions to treat respiratory symptoms of COVID-19. e) For all prescriptions of albuterol inhalers, pharmacists shall conduct a

---

64 https://portal.ct.gov/-/media/Departments-and-Agencies/DPH/Facility-Licensing--Investigations/Blast-Faxes/Blast-Fax-2020-29-Updated-Guidance-for-COVID-19.pdf?la=en

65 https://www.oplc.nh.gov/pharmacy/documents/dhhs-emergency-order-04-03-2020.pdf

prospective drug utilization review to ensure adherence to asthma controller or maintenance medications, and counsel patients that are non-compliant and over-utilizing rescue inhalers. 2. This Order shall remain in effect until the State of Emergency declared by the Governor is terminated, or this Order is rescinded, whichever shall happen first.

New York:[66]

No pharmacist shall dispense hydroxychloroquine or chloroquine except when written as prescribed for an FDA-approved indication; or as part of a state approved clinical trial related to COVID-19 for a patient who has tested positive for COVID-19, with such test result documented as part of the prescription. No other experimental or prophylactic use shall be permitted, and any permitted prescription is limited to one fourteen day prescription with no refills.

Oregon:[67]

Updated 6/15/2020

Oregon's pharmacy board put out a new rule on 6/15:

"Prescription orders for chloroquine or hydroxychloroquine for the prevention or treatment of

---

66 https://www.governor.ny.gov/news/no-20210-continuing-temporary-suspension-and-modification-laws-relating-disaster-emergency

67 https://secure.sos.state.or.us/oard/viewReceiptPDF.action?filingRsn=44884

COVID-19 infection may only be dispensed if written for a patient enrolled in a clinical trial by an authorized investigator."

And the board cites the FDA revocation of the EUA:

NEED FOR THE RULE(S): On 6/15/2020, the FDA revoked the emergency use authorization (EUA) that allowed for chloroquine phosphate and hydroxychloroquine sulfate donated to the Strategic National Stockpile to be used to treat certain hospitalized patients with COVID-19 when a clinical trial was unavailable, or participation in a clinical trial was not feasible. The agency determined that the legal criteria for issuing an EUA are no longer met. Based on its ongoing analysis of the EUA and emerging scientific data, the FDA determined that chloroquine and hydroxychloroquine are unlikely to be effective in treating COVID-19 for the authorized uses in the EUA. Additionally, in light of ongoing serious cardiac adverse events and other potential serious side effects, the known and potential benefits of chloroquine and hydroxychloroquine no longer outweigh the known and potential risks for the authorized use. Furthermore, hydroxychloroquine continues to remain on the FDA's drug shortage list.

It bears repeating that to be FDA approved, a drug has to go through years of testing. To be FDA approved for 65 years is an overwhelming testimonial to a drug's safety and efficacy. There is no need for additional government intrusion.

Only a handful of states let doctors continue to be doctors. Florida did not get involved in the politicization of a drug. Florida spoke loudly and clearly by adding nothing additional to the already massive amounts of drug regulations by the Governor, the state medical board and the state pharmacy board.

Why Is HCQ Being Maligned?

COVID-19 is an acronym for SARS-CoV-2. It is so named because it turns out there was a SARS-CoV-1. Reading the scientific literature related to the first SARS is so eerily similar that excerpts are copy/pasted on the next page. In 2002 there was a new coronavirus, originating in China, which rapidly spread to dozens of countries, within a few months, leading to worldwide efforts to contain it. The scientists discovered that CQ had a strong antiviral effect on this SARS-CoV virus, whether the CQ was used before or after infection. It was concluded that CQ had both prophylactic and therapeutic use.

The study "Chloroquine is a Potent Inhibitor of SARS Coronavirus Infection and Spread" by Vincent, Bergeron, Benjannet, et. al., was published by the official publication of the National Institutes of Health when Dr. Fauci was NIH Director:[68] Given that CQ was demonstrated to be very effective against a 78% identical coronavirus less than 15 years ago during a very similar situation, it is very curious that there was a multinational effort to restrict it starting in mid-January. (CQ is a precursor to the more modern HCQ. We now use HCQ in the USA. But studies of CQ are as reliable as studies of HCQ.)

On January 13, 2020 France quietly changed the status of

---

[68] https://www.ncbi.nlm.nih.gov/pmc/articles/PMC1232869/

HCQ from its years long over-the-counter status to "List II poisonous substance."[69] This was an unprecedented demotion. And in the USA: "Dr. Anthony Fauci said Wednesday that data shows HCQ is not an effective agent for the coronavirus, disputing use of the drug to fight the deadly virus even as President Donald Trump touts it as a potential cure."[70]

It is unclear when Dr. Fauci came to believe the opposite of what the NIH published when he was the NIH Director. What we do know is that 70,000-100,000 excess American lives have been lost due to lack of access to HCQ. So why did a medication that had been over the counter for decades, suddenly but quietly get pulled from the shelves, in the midst of a pandemic, due to a virus that is so similar it shares a name?

It is well known that newly patented drugs can be extremely profitable if there is demand and no other supply. The demand for Gilead's Remdisivir, which is used **late** in the disease, obviously will plummet if the disease is stopped by HCQ **early**. Remdisivir is sold for $3200-$5700 per treatment and the federal government has already purchased all or most of it.[71] The generic HCQ is ~$10 per treatment.

69 https://www.legifrance.gouv.fr/jo_pdf.do?id=JORFTEXT000041400024

70 https://www.cnn.com/2020/05/27/politics/anthony-fauci-hydroxychloroquine-trump-cnntv/index.html

71 https://omnij.org/Gilead:_Twenty one_billion_reasons_to_discredit_hydroxychloroquine_(ORIGINAL_ARTICLE)

Background

Severe acute respiratory syndrome (SARS) is caused by a newly discovered coronavirus (SARS-CoV). No effective prophylactic or post-exposure therapy is currently available.

Results

We report, however, that chloroquine has strong antiviral effects on SARS-CoV infection of primate cells. These inhibitory effects are observed when the cells are treated with the drug either before or after exposure to the virus, suggesting both prophylactic and therapeutic advantage. In addition to the well-known functions of chloroquine such as elevations of endosomal pH, the drug appears to interfere with terminal glycosylation of the cellular receptor, angiotensin-converting enzyme 2. This may negatively influence the virus-receptor binding and abrogate the infection, with further ramifications by the elevation of vesicular pH, resulting in the inhibition of infection and spread of SARS CoV at clinically admissible concentrations.

Background

Severe acute respiratory syndrome (SARS) is an emerging disease that was first reported in Guangdong Province, China, in late 2002. The disease rapidly spread to at least 30 countries within months of its first appearance, and concerted worldwide efforts led to the identification of the etiological agent as SARS coronavirus (SARS-CoV), a novel member of the family *Coronaviridae* [1]. Complete genome

Discussion

We have identified chloroquine as an effective antiviral agent for SARS-CoV in cell culture conditions, as evidenced by its inhibitory effect when the drug was added prior to infection or after the initiation and establishment of infection. The fact that chloroquine exerts an antiviral effect during pre- and post-infection conditions suggest that it is likely to have both prophylactic and therapeutic advantages. Recently, Keyaerts et al. [21] reported the antiviral properties of chloroquine and identified that the drug affects SARS-CoV replication in cell culture, as evidenced by quantitative RT-PCR. Taken together with the findings of Keyaerts et al. [21], our analysis provides further evidence that chloroquine is effective against SARS-CoV Frankfurt and Urbani strains. We have provided evidence that chloroquine is effective in preventing SARS-CoV infection in cell culture if the drug is added to the cells 24 h prior to infection. In addition, chloroquine was significantly effective even when the drug was added 3–5 h after infection, suggesting an antiviral effect even after the establishment of infection. Since similar results were obtained by NH_4Cl treatment of Vero E6 cells, the underlying mechanism(s) of action of these drugs might be similar.

Conclusion

Chloroquine, a relatively safe, effective and cheap drug used for treating many human diseases including malaria, amoebiasis and human immunodeficiency virus is effective in inhibiting the infection and spread of SARS CoV in cell culture. The fact that the drug has significant inhibitory antiviral effect when the susceptible cells were treated either prior to or after infection suggests a possible prophylactic and therapeutic use.

Implications for the USA if restrictions on HCQ are not lifted immediately.

The safety of HCQ is so well established that it should have been over the counter decades ago, and in fact that is how it is in much of the world. The process to move a medication from prescription to over the counter in America is typically driven by a pharmaceutical company that has a profit motive: is a safe, well-established drug more profitable, at this time, over the counter? That is how drugs such as Zantac, Pepcid, Zyrtec, Allegra, Aleve, Benadryl, Minoxidil and nicotine patches and others came to be over the counter.

HCQ is safe but there's no profit motive to move it to over the counter, as there have been no general usage indication in America. It would languish on the shelves. So it sits in the armamentarium of prescription drugs, and quite frankly, no one gave it much thought prior to this pandemic. However, the landscape has changed, and now there is an urgent impetus to make it readily available to the American people.

It is interesting to note that many over the counter drugs, probably the majority, are less safe than HCQ. For example Tylenol, and aspirin are listed as more risky.[72] Most doctors would attest to the frequent problems people have with Motrin/Ibuprofen/Aleve. Tylenol toxicity is the most common reason for liver transplant in the USA and anti-inflammatories account for an enormous number of GI bleeds/pain/distress.

---

72 https://www.thedenverchannel.com/news/national/these-are-the-50-most-dangerous-drugs-on-the-market

If the disinformation campaign regarding HCQ weren't so complete, from the scientific journals, to the media, to the state medical boards to the FDA, this would not really matter. Individual physicians who are innovators and early adopters would have moved first, prescribing HCQ off-label, just as physicians already do 20% of the time, and it would have caught on rapidly. However, the disinformation campaign blocked off-label use, and now we are in a pandemic with a safe and effective drug that doctors inclined to prescribe and patients inclined to take, cannot access.

As a result, not only are patients not being treated promptly, effectively, and safely, some patients die. And as the fear of the pandemic has overtaken the virus itself and it is impossible to change public and physician opinion quickly enough to save lives, we must make the medication available to the public directly.

Dr. Harvey Risch, MD, PhD, Professor of Epidemiology at Yale School of Public Health and published in affiliation with the Johns Hopkins Bloomberg School of Public Health.[73] Dr. Risch who has 39,779 citations on Google Scholar, notes that:[74]

> "US cumulative deaths through July 15 are 140,000. Had we permitted HCQ use liberally, we would have saved half, 70,000 and it is very possible we could have saved 3/4, 105,000."

---

73 https://www.aspph.org/yale-dr-harvey-risch-wins-50000-ruth-leff-siegel-award/

74 Interview with the author July 15, 2020

It is relevant that the problem that the USA has with accessing hydroxychloroquine is a first-world problem. Curiously the people who *cannot* get HCQ typically live in first-world democracies. Speaking generally, HCQ or its progenitor CQ, was freely available over the counter in most of the world Africa, Asia, South America, even Canada and Mexico, prior to Covid. Long before President Trump endorsed HCQ on March 20, 2020, the drug was quietly removed from pharmacy shelves in Canada and it was banned outright in France. These two actions were taken in January 2020. It is speculation as to why but one must consider who benefits if HCQ is not accessible.

It cannot be overlooked that right now, all over the world, patients who want to buy HCQ simply do. Iran, Costa Rica, Italy, Panama; many others. Here is a photograph of a typical pharmacy in Indonesia taken on July 16, 2020.[75]

---

75 @Smackenziekerr July 17, 2020

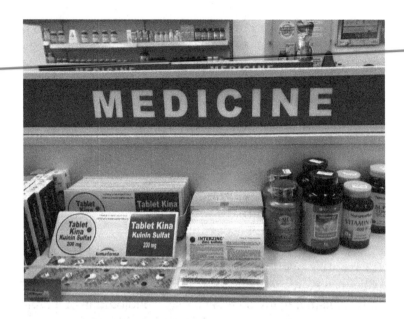

No matter the reason, there is an obvious relationship between access to HCQ and mortality rates from Covid-19. While it is true that such a relationship does not prove cause/effect, but it is also true that it would be lunacy to assume no relationship.[76]

---

76 AAPS vs. FDA https://aapsonline.org/judicial/aaps-v-fda-hcq-6-2-2020.pdf

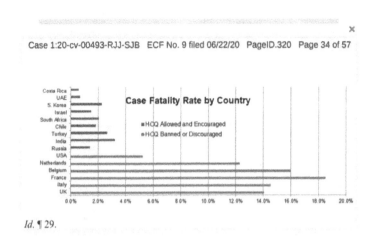

Case 1:20-cv-00493-RJJ-SJB ECF No. 9 filed 06/22/20 PageID.320 Page 34 of 57

Id. ¶ 29.

Country by country data is also available and access to HCQ is strongly linked to lower mortality.[77] We can see that even very poor countries have much lower case fatality rates than wealthy countries, which of course, is typically the opposite of what we would expect of a respiratory disease that could end up in an ICU admission. Kazakhstan, Bangladesh, Senegal, Pakistan, Serbia, Nigeria, Turkey, Ukraine, Honduras … the list goes on. Wealthier democracies or countries with especially abusive HCQ protocols such as are doing terribly: Ireland, Canada, Spain, The Netherlands, UK, Belgium, France ... Of note, Italy and Spain switched mid-stream and now HCQ is easily available.

---

77 https://docs.google.com/spreadsheets/d/14GUXRGzNTV1BUgY6xvpFM-fYDTxXvKCUSUrTThnwwfh8/edit#gid=0

Country	Mortality : # of deaths	# of cases	CFR old	Deaths per l	HCQ policy	As of June 21, 2020 - numbers fr
Qatar	94	86488	0.11%		encourages HCQ Qatar's health minister says country uses HCQ and	
Bahrain	60	21,331	0.28%		encourages HCQ: Bahrain among first countries to use Hydroxychloro	
Oman	128	28,566	0.45%	2	encourages HCQ: Oman has approved the antimalaria drug, HCQ, as	
Costa Rica	12	2,127	0.56%		encourages HCQ use	
Belarus	343	57936	0.59%		encourages HCQ: Sandoz will donate potential effective drug for treati	
UAE	301	44,533	0.68%	31	encourages HCQ use: UAE says it is successfully treating patients wit	
Kazakhstan	118	16779	0.70%		encourages HCQ: Pakistan donated 700,000 chloroquine tablets to Ka	
Saudi Arabia	1230	154,233	0.80%		"Saudi Arabia's treatment plan from March which shows HCQ use dat	
Bangladesh	1425	108775	1.31%		encourages HCQ: Bangladesh recommends controversial drugs for C	
Russia	8002	576,952	1.39%	55	Russia recommended PrEP use of HCQ: Post contact prevention in in	
Malaysia	121	8556	1.41%		encourages HCQ: "Malaysia Finds Hydroxychloroquine Can Slow Cou	
Senegal	82	5,783	1.42%		encourages HCQ use, Senegal will continue use of HCQ + azithromyc	
Israel	305	20,633	1.48%	33	encourages HCQ: PM Netanyahu thanks Modi for donation of HCQ	
Chile	4295	236748	1.81%	234	" In Chile, a centralized national Protocol was made in which both Pub	
Pakistan	3382	171,666	1.97%		"Pakistan asks India for Hydroxychloroquine to combat coronavirus ou	
South Africa	1877	92,681	2.03%	33	" here in South Africa HCQ is used widely for malaria so the last three	
Serbia	260	12,803	2.03%		Serbian and Bosnian drugmakers Galenika and Zada Pharmaceutical	
Morocco	213	9,839	2.16%		encourages: "Morocco to Receive 6 Million Hydroxychloroquine Table	
S. Korea	280	12,421	2.25%	5	encourages HCQ use	
Argentina	992	41,204	2.41%		Several reports of patients in Argentina noting they received HCQ	
Nigeria	506	19,808	2.55%		"Nigerian authorities say they will continue to use hydroxychloroquine	
Turkey	4927	186493	2.64%	59	encouraged HCQ use	
Ukraine	994	35,825	2.77%		encourages HCQ use	
Honduras	358	12,306	2.91%		"the Honduran government assured that hydroxychloroquine will cont	
Peru	7861	251338	3.13%		Peru will continue to use the controversial drug hydroxychloroquine to	
Czechia	336	10,448	3.22%		Czech Health Ministry permits temporary use of hydroxychloroquine to	
India	13277	411727	3.22%	10	encourages HCQ use	
Colombia	2126	65633	3.24%		"Hydroxychloroquine and Chloroquine Can Be Used to Treat Covid-19	
Philippines	1150	29,400	3.91%		Makati Medical Center (MMC) is using Hcq-Az plus zinc and Vitamin C	

Egypt		2106	53756	3.92%		Egyptian Health Minister on Hydroxychloroquine: "We put it in the trea
Portugal		1528	38,841	3.93%		Patients in Portugal with Covid-19 can be treated with malaria and ebc
Austria		688	17,323	3.97%		" Malaria drug is used in Austria" hospitalized pts
Poland		1346	31,620	4.26%		Some use in Poland was noted March 13
Brazil		50,056	1,070,139	4.68%		asked US for HCQ late in the process, poor distribution, isolated use
Germany		8961	191,216	4.69%		only 13% of doctors in Germany said they would prescribe HCQ
Iran		9,507	202,584	4.69%		not clear
Denmark	5	600	12,391	4.94%		"hydroxychloroquine in Denmark can only be prescribed by hospital do
USA		121,980	2,330,578	5.23%	369	blocked HCQ use (a few brave physicians use it), isolated use where a
Japan	6	952	17,799	5.35%		Hydroxychloroquine usage amongst COVID-19 treaters is 7% in Japa
China		4634	83,378	5.56%		didn't know about HCQ initially
Greece		190	3,256	5.84%		Greece has resumed production of chloroquine to treat cases of coron
Switzerland		1956	31,243	6.26%		"hospitalised Covid-19 patients" i.e. too late
Ireland	7	1715	25,374	6.76%		Apparently HCQ was frowned upon in Ireland
Canada	8	8,410	101019	8.33%		very anti-HCQ leadership.
Ecuador	8	4156	49,731	8.36%		At least one city in Ecuador used it reported success
Sweden	9	5053	56,043	9.02%		April 6: Several Swedish Hospitals Have Stopped Using Chloroquine
Spain	10	28322	293018	9.67%	606	Hydroxychloroquine usage amongst COVID-19 treaters is 72% in Spa
Algeria		837	8,324	10.06%		Dr. Idir Bitam reports that in Algeria of 170 people treated with HCQ +
Mexico	12	20,781	175,202	11.86%		very anti-Trump leadership, poor distibution
Netherlands	12	6089	49,502	12.30%	365	some hospitals used HCQ, but early use apparently discouraged. prot
UK	15	42589	303110	14.05%	628	only 13% of UK physicians said they used it
Italy	15	34,610	238,275	14.53%	573	did not initially know about HCQ (eventually adopted in some areas) a
Belgium	15	9,696	60550	16.01%	837	Belgium used HCQ "for the sickest coronavirus patients."
France	18	29,633	160,093	18.51%	454	France banned HCQ

The limitation or outright ban on HCQ worldwide has begun to crack. It will soon collapse because the evidence of its safety and efficacy is so overwhelming. The countries that have less flexibility to tolerate fatal policies have already reversed themselves. South of us, Honduras, Panama, Costa Rica have, or earlier had, made HCQ available. Brazil is trying but faces many of the same political problems as the USA. Some countries have started going door to door to facilitate its availability.[78]

In Honduras their national policy now is: "The patient that presents for the first time to a First Level of Care facility, if so, treatment should be started with: Acetaminophen, Hydroxychloroquine 400 every 12 hours, Ivermectin, Azithromycin, Zinc ..."[79]

Puede que el paciente se presente por primera vez a un Establecimiento del Primer Nivel de Atención, si es así se debe iniciar tratamiento con:

- Acetaminofén 500mg V.O. c/6 hrs en caso de fiebre.
- Hidroxicloroquina 400 mg V.O. c/12 hrs primer día, luego 400 mg /día x 5 días
- Ivermectina 200 µg/kg día x 5 días.
- Azitromicina 500 mg V.O. /día x 5 días
- Zinc 100 mg V.O. c/día x 5 días.
- Colchicina* 1 mg V.O primera dosis, luego 0.5 mg V.O c/12 hrs hasta que valores inflamatorios disminuyan por al menos 2 días consecutivos.
- Prednisona 1mg/kg/día V.O x 7 días
- Apixabán* 5mg V.O. c/12 hrs o Rivaroxabán* 20 mg V.O. c/día con la comida x 14 días
- Autoaislamiento en el Hogar con vigilancia médica.
- **Pronación voluntaria**

* Se debe ajustar dosis en pacientes con insuficiencia renal y adultos mayores.

---

78 Conversation author had with Dr. Sanchez, head of FDA Honduras July 10, 2020. https://www.arsa.gob.hn/

79 Conversation author had with Maria Dolores Aguero Ministra De Relaciones Exteriores July 9, 2020

Panama reversed course regarding HCQ and many countries in South and Central America are following suit:[80]

> Evaluating new evidence around the therapeutic options for COVID-19, specifically the use of HCQ and the Lancet journal withdrawing its publication on this topic. The Ministry of Health communicates that Circular No. 118-DGSP is null and void, establishing directives for immediate compliance regarding the use of HCQ and / or azithromycin. Leaving the therapeutic option for prescription according to medical criteria. Soon we will be sending a treatment guide for Covid-19 patients.

---

80 Dr. Luis Francisco Sucre Mejia – Ministro de Salud

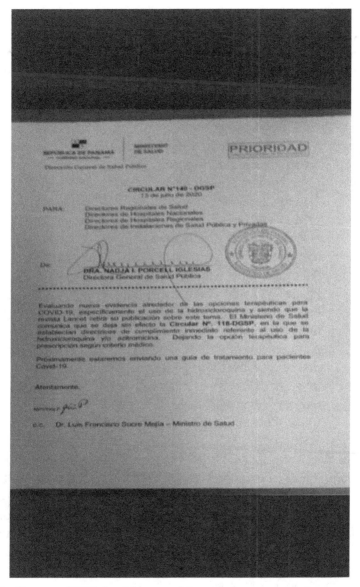

In France, HCQ had been sold over the counter for many years, but on January 15, 2020, then Health minister Buzyn reclassified it as "list II of poisonous substances." Three days after Trump endorsed it, the next Health Minister Veran said that HCQ was only to be used for severely ill hospitalized patients and could not be used early or prophylaxis use. Then two months later he terminated using it at all. All this time, esteemed virologist Professor Raoult continued his clinical trials and in his hospitals the mortality rate was 0.52% compared to the rest of France 19.12%. Because this was so mishandled, resulting in so many unnecessary deaths, the former French Prime Minister and two Ministers of Health are now being criminally investigated.[81]

> Former French Prime Minister, health ministers to be investigated for pandemic response"
> A French court will investigate former French Prime Minister Edouard Philippe and two health ministers following complaints about the government's handling of the coronavirus pandemic, Prosecutor General François Molins said today. Philippe, former Health Minister Agnès Buzyn and outgoing Health Minister Olivier Véran will have to respond to accusations of abstaining from fighting a disaster.

In The Netherlands, Dr. R. Elens, has filed suit due to his being blocked from prescribing HCQ, which is contrary to his lifelong practice as a physician.[82] He was sanctioned and could face a fine of Euro150,000. He filed this petition to clarify the status of HCQ and will pursue to The Hague if necessary as a crime against humanity.

---

81 https://www.politico.eu/article/former-french-pm-health-ministers-to-be-investigated-for-pandemic-response/

82 https://zelfzorgcovid19.nl/wp-content/uploads/2020/06/voornemen-off-label-gebruik.pdf

As in all battles of good vs. evil, when America falters, the world collapses.

Conclusion:

This white paper is to draw the reader's attention to the indisputable safety of HCQ, remarkable efficacy of HCQ against SARS-CoV-2, and the worldwide political storm that has resulted in its use being restricted. We speak in support of it being made available over the counter in the USA due to the inability of Americans to access it, whether they need it for treatment or to manage their fear.[83]

The virus is known to be asymptomatic or mild the vast majority of the time, but in people with multiple co-morbid conditions, rarely it can be deadly. Because so much was unknown in the beginning, the most cautious approach was taken. However, now that we know the facts, it has proven impossible to dislodge the fear that was implemented.

At this time, disinformation and therefore resultant fear have a firmer grip on Americans than reality. And thus Americans who need a life-saving medication cannot get it either due to their own physicians' reluctance, their pharmacies regulating against the same, their state medical boards threats, the media disinformation, and/or due to certain sectors of the federal government's own anti-HCQ statements.

Some people question if making HCQ over the counter would change anything, as there has been such negative coverage. The answer is like all things in life: there are in-

---

83 https://www.wsj.com/articles/notable-quotable-fear-for-our-children-11594854726?st=qb7dqvvapgd7s2z&reflink=article_email_share

novators, early adopters, early majority, late majority and laggards. What has gone wrong in this instance is that innovators and early adopters have been stymied. Once people are free again to make their own choices, they will, and society will normalize over about a month.

Once Americans know they can buy a safe, cheap, generic, life-saving medication, should they need it, calm and rationality can be restored, not just to America, but throughout the world. A person who suffers from an occasional migraine headache but who has the migraine medicine at home or in her pocket, in case she needs it, is a person who feels safe and comfortable going about her daily routine. If she does not have that prescription, she may limit herself a lot or a little, and either way, she is fearful of what is around the corner.

At the very least, the efficacy "assassination" of HCQ must be reversed immediately. Doctors must be able to prescribe HCQ as a treatment and as a prophylaxis. It is absolutely unacceptable that doctors are not being able to communicate responsibly and with compassion with their patients. That must be remedied. Period.

Americans do not need to be afraid. Instead, they need to be empowered. Their physicians should not be prevented from upholding their Hippocratic Oath and healing their patients. Instead, they must be permitted to practices sound and safe medicine. Patients and their doctors must be able to discuss the options for optimal care and treatment and the patient-physician relationship must take precedent.

ABOUT THE AUTHOR

Simone Gold, MD, JD, FABEM, is a board-certified emergency physician. She graduated from Chicago Medical School before attending Stanford University Law School to earn her Juris Doctorate degree. She completed her residency in Emergency Medicine at Stony Brook University Hospital in New York. Dr. Gold worked in Washington, D.C. for the Surgeon General, as well as for the Chairman of the Labor and Human Resources Committee. She works as an emergency physician on the frontlines. Her clinical work serves all Americans: from urban-inner city, to suburban and the Native American population. She writes on a number of policy issues relating to law and medicine. She always leads with the facts.